The Woman Who Cured Cancer

The Story of Cancer Pioneer
Virginia Livingston-Wheeler, M.D.,
and the Discovery of the
Cancer-Causing Microbe

EDMOND G. ADDEO

T0273535

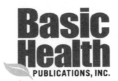

Basic
Health
PUBLICATIONS, INC.

The information contained in this book is based upon the research and personal and professional experiences of the author. All examples and quotes herein are composites of many people and do not refer to any one particular person. The names used were made up and do not reflect any real names of people connected to the symptoms or examples used. It is not intended as a substitute for consulting with your physician or other healthcare provider. Any attempt to diagnose and treat an illness should be done under the direction of a healthcare professional.

The publisher does not advocate the use of any particular healthcare protocol but believes the information in this book should be available to the public. The publisher and author are not responsible for any adverse effects or consequences resulting from the use of the suggestions, preparations, or procedures discussed in this book. Should the reader have any questions concerning the appropriateness of any procedures or preparation mentioned, the author and the publisher strongly suggest consulting a professional healthcare advisor.

Basic Health Publications, Inc.
28812 Top of the World Drive
Laguna Beach, CA 92651
949-715-7327 • www.basichealthpub.com

Library of Congress Cataloging-in-Publication Data
Addeo, Edmond G., author.
    The woman who cured cancer : the story of cancer pioneer Virginia Livingston-Wheeler, M.D., and the discovery of the cancer-causing microbe / Edmond G. Addeo.
        p. ; cm.
    Follow-up to: The conquest of cancer : vaccines and diet / Virginia Livingston-Wheeler and Edmond G. Addeo. 1984.
    Includes bibliographical references and index.
    ISBN 978-1-59120-372-8
    I. Title.
    [DNLM: 1. Livingston-Wheeler, Virginia 2. Neoplasms—microbiology. 3. Neoplasms—therapy. 4. Physicians, Women—Biography. 5. Neoplasms—etiology. WZ 100]
    RC265.5
    616.99'40092—dc23
    [B]
                                                              2014023973

Editor: Cheryl Hirsch
Typesetting/Book design: Gary A. Rosenberg • www.thebookcouple.com
Cover design: Mike Stromberg

Printed in the United States of America

10   9   8   7   6   5   4   3   2   1

Contents

This book is dedicated to the memory of
Dr. Virginia Livingston-Wheeler (1906–1990),
to agent Bill Gladstone, who brought us together
in 1982 for the eventual publishing of *The Conquest
of Cancer* in 1984, and to John O'Melveny Woods,
who has kept Dr. Virginia's memory alive and who
inspired and encouraged this new work.

Foreword

It is with great pleasure that I introduce this amazing book, a follow-up to *The Conquest of Cancer: Vaccines and Diet* (1984). Virginia Livingston-Wheeler, M.D., was a close friend and inspiration to me. When I first met Dr. Virginia in 1981, I was senior editor for Harcourt Brace Jovanovich Publishing based in San Diego, California. I was responsible for finding brilliant authors with manuscripts and book ideas worthy of publication. I cannot remember how I was introduced to Dr. Virginia, but I remember sitting in the waiting room at her clinic thinking how extraordinary her accomplishments were. She had not only been the first female medical intern in the city of New York but had pioneered alternative treatments to cancer and had saved hundreds if not thousands of lives. She had been the first medical doctor to see the connection between diet and cancer and had developed specific treatment modalities for patients whom other doctors in many cases had given up on as non-treatable.

When I walked into Dr. Virginia's office I was expecting a taciturn or at least a stern encounter with an "all business focus." As it turned out that was not the case at all. Dr. Virginia, although approaching seventy at the time, was a lively, witty, and refreshing woman who exuded the youthful enthusiasm of a woman half her age. She asked me astute questions about how Harcourt would publish her book and why I rather than another editor should be granted the rights. My responses must have been adequate, since a few weeks later we signed a deal memo for Harcourt to publish her book. At the time, as senior editor and editorial director of Harcourt West Coast, I had the authority to sign contracts without the approval of Peter Jovanovich, to whom I reported as the head of the trade division of the company.

Much to my surprise and disappointment when the actual contract forms were presented for Peter's signature, Peter called me and explained that he was going to have to overrule me and cancel this contract. Apparently, Harcourt was the publisher of a trade magazine for the poultry industry, and of course Dr. Virginia's manuscript was quite critical of the chicken industry, documenting links between the way chickens were being raised and prepared for consumers and high cancer rates in those consuming chicken regularly from these sources. Harcourt's significant financial investment in the trade magazine was more important to the company than publishing Dr. Virginia's book. I protested, but to no avail, and had to explain to Dr. Virginia that we would not be able to work together after all. I did promise that I would check as a personal favor with editors and colleagues at other publishing houses and find an alternative publisher.

My initial calls to other publishers were not immediately fruitful. They wanted to see more of the manuscript, which was not yet written, and they wanted a complete proposal, which Dr. Virginia had not prepared. I had been able to meet directly with her and have my questions answered, not in a proposal, but in my personal review of Dr. Virginia's clinic and interviews with her staff. I explained the obstacles to Dr. Virginia and left it to her to have her staff create a full book proposal.

As one of John Lennon's songs says, "Life is what happens when you are busy making other plans." For reasons unrelated to Dr. Virginia, a few months after Harcourt rejected the opportunity to publish *The Conquest of Cancer,* I found myself no longer with Harcourt but setting up my own company, Waterside Productions Inc., to be a documentary and, eventually, feature film production company. I left Harcourt in November 1981, and as I was creating my film company I started getting calls from other authors such as David Loye, whose book *The Sphinx and the Rainbow* (1984) I had signed before departing Harcourt. David and other authors were contacting me to let me know that after I left Harcourt they had received notices that their contracts were being cancelled. Harcourt did not have a replacement editor who truly understood many of the cutting-edge titles I had signed prior to my departure and exercised the termination clauses that allowed the authors to keep the signing portion of their advances but not to proceed to publication.

I knew I had to assist these authors, none of whom had literary agents at the time, and set up a sideline for Waterside to serve not just as a film production company but also as a literary agency. In doing this I remembered that Dr. Virginia still had not had her staff produce the book proposal that was required to pitch the book to other publishers. The universe supports positive action. My action in taking on literary agenting as part of Waterside produced a flood of queries from writers wanting to either have their own manuscript placed or seeking work writing or ghostwriting for others.

One of these queries was from Ed Addeo. Ed had significant writing credits and seemed an ideal person to connect with Dr. Virginia since it was apparent that Dr. Virginia's staff was much too busy saving lives to write book proposals. When I approached Ed with the idea of working with Dr. Virginia, he was ecstatic. He knew of her work and greatly admired her accomplishments. I called Dr. Virginia and introduced her to Ed, who promptly flew to San Diego from his home in Mill Valley, and the rest is history.

Ed created a wonderful book proposal and a few weeks later we had a contract offer from Franklin Watts, a major New York publishing house. This was in 1982 and as it turned out was the very first book ever agented by me and Waterside. I was overjoyed to have finally fulfilled my promise to help Dr. Virginia reach the large audience her research deserved. I knew that *The Conquest of Cancer* would save lives and I now know it has. Two years later her book was published.

Along the way Dr. Virginia became a great friend, inviting me to amazing parties held at her home in La Jolla, California. She even allowed me to use her spacious home for the wedding reception for my marriage. Dr. Virginia always referred to me as her publisher when she introduced me to her friends. In the beginning I would explain that I was actually just her agent and not actually her publisher. Eventually, since Dr. Virginia continued to insist in introducing me as her publisher, I stopped explaining the difference between being her agent and being her publisher.

Life is a journey and we never know exactly when bumps and obstacles will appear. If you or someone in your family has been diagnosed with cancer you know what a severe bump that is. My mother died of cancer at the relatively young age of sixty-two. She was already past treatment, having had radiation and chemotherapy before I had had the chance to introduce her to Dr. Virginia only two months before she passed. I often think that she might have survived had Dr. Virginia's book been published a few years earlier. May this book prevent others from dying prematurely.

With all best wishes for health and happiness,

William Gladstone
Founder and President, Waterside Productions,
Cardiff-by-the-Sea, California

Preface

First of all, the word "cured" in the title needs to be explained. I know full well that the word sets off all kinds of warning lights in the medical community. Indeed, the words "quack" and "charlatan" and "alternative" and a host of related terms usually ensue. This book should actually be titled *The Woman Who Put Cancer into Permanent Remission* to mollify professional critics. But that's too cumbersome for a title.

Second, I purposely chose to keep the word "cured" in order to get people's attention. Virginia Livingston-Wheeler, M.D., did, indeed, cure patients of their cancer with the vaccine she developed. As she was wont to say, "My patients' names are in phone books, not on gravestones." In fact, there has been so much good news about new cancer vaccines that the reader deserves to hear it in the first chapter before we go into the history of the Livingston cancer vaccine's development in San Diego.

In this book, you'll read about some of the other good news about cancer treatments being published every day. These "news updates" have been included to familiarize the reader in general about various current cancer treatments, research projects, and nutritional developments that seem to be progressions of Dr. Virginia's treatments. I am tempted to call them "corroborations," because several of these news subjects were once considered outrageous and generated ridicule for her clinic but are accepted medical practice today. The updates are brief because I encourage readers to use the Internet to read the entire story of the scientific development.

But here is the best news of all and one of the chief reasons for writing this book: the cancer vaccine developed by Dr. Virginia forty years ago at her clinic in San Diego is still available today! John Majnarich, Ph.D., the biochemist who made the vaccine for her clinic and who is the co-holder of the patent, is still making it in his laboratory in Redmond, Washington, for hundreds of other physicians and surgeons ever since Dr. Virginia died. (In the Resources section at the end of this book I'll tell you how to reach his lab.) Also, a new Livingston Foundation has been formed, which is committed to keeping the knowledge and ideas promulgated and practiced by Dr. Virginia Livingston-Wheeler in the public domain for future generations. In this respect, all of her work, published and unpublished, as well as videos and other archival material, is available at www.LivingstonFoundation.com free of charge to anyone who would like to learn of her amazing work and discoveries. Additionally, the website is dynamically updated regarding the latest discoveries in autogenous vaccines and related fields of research and, if appropriate, will give referrals to physicians around the world who administer the Livingston vaccine and Dr. Virginia's other protocols in the treatment of other autoimmune diseases.

As mentioned, the vaccine is "autogenous," which means it isn't a "one-size-fits-all" product but instead is made from each patient's individual tumor cells. Hence, it doesn't require Food and Drug Administration (FDA) approval. This is the first question I usually get in my lectures and interviews, especially by medical doctors. When I explain why the vaccine does *not* need FDA approval, they seem satisfied, albeit still skeptical.

The second question I get is, "If it's so effective, why doesn't the medical community know about it?" And the answer to that is twofold: 1) they *do* know about it, but they don't want *you* to know about it, because 2) if you were making trillions of dollars a year peddling chemotherapy drugs and radiation apparatus, would *you* want to see a $1,000 vaccine come along?

So, read on. No one needs to die of cancer. Dr. Virginia's story will tell you why.

1

The Vaccine Works!

Over the years since her death in 1990, physicians around the country who knew about Dr. Virginia Livingston-Wheeler's work or who heard through old-fashioned word-of-mouth about her autogenous vaccines have been using the vaccines to treat their patients. To me, the remarkable thing about this is that it is practicing mainstream physicians and surgeons who are using the vaccines, not "alternative" clinics or fringe-credible practitioners. These doctors obviously believe that the vaccines have some beneficial effect and are not hesitant to administer them. The trouble is, they won't admit it for fear of losing their licenses (of this, more later). I believe their use of the vaccine may go as far back as 1991, when a *New England Journal of Medicine* article determined that the Livingston protocol for cancer (vaccine, vegetarian diet, high dosages of vitamin A, and other modalities) was no worse than standard treatment, and it probably made a lasting impression on the medical community.

Greg's Story

In one recent case, Greg H., a fifty-nine-year-old man who had undergone three surgeries for brain cancer (glioblastoma), had been told that any further surgery would be meaningless and that he had only six months to live. Gliobastoma is rare but is one of the deadliest types of brain tumor. He had been going to regular gym workouts when one day he noticed in the mirror that the right side of his face was sagging, as if he'd had a stroke. Later that afternoon his head started flopping as if his neck muscles had given out, and he ran to his doctor.

The doctor immediately sent him to the emergency room where he was examined and sent to a prominent local hospital for a brain scan, which revealed a tumor that was 1.2 centimeters (0.5 inches) long by 0.3 centimeters (0.1 inches) thick. This was in November 2010. He was given six weeks of radiation and chemotherapy, but by February 2011 he had a recurrence of symptoms and a second surgery. Further radiation and chemo only led to a third surgery, until he was finally told further treatment was useless and he had a maximum of six months to live.

Despondent and desperate for alternatives, Greg was told about the Livingston vaccine's availability by a friend, and began taking it. To make a long story short, when I interviewed him in preparation for this book he told me that a recent magnetic resonance imaging (MRI) scan showed that the tumor had completely disappeared. He now has an MRI every two months and a follow-up vaccine shot once a month, and has remained clear of any evidence of cancer.

Rolph's Story

I have a close friend, a retired oral surgeon, who was diagnosed a few years ago with chronic lymphocytic leukemia (CLL), a cancer of the blood-forming tissues (bone marrow, lymph system, or spleen). Rolph underwent chemotherapy with a combination of drugs that nearly killed him. He lost weight dramatically, his energy plummeted, his scalp itched continually, and he developed lesions on his back, boils on his legs, nasal discharges, aching bones, a persistent cough, and was always tired but could not sleep.

I had lunch in June 2012 with Rolph and a mutual friend. When Rolph got up to shuffle to the men's room, I commented to the friend that I thought he would be dead by Thanksgiving. He looked terrible. His face was ash gray, he was thin, and he could hardly walk, steadying himself on the backs of chairs as he went. This was a man who loved golf, skiing, and once climbed Mt. Everest.

That afternoon I took Rolph aside and told him about the Livingston vaccine's availability from a laboratory in Redmond, Washington. Rolph was skeptical (as so many are!) but I insisted that, as a doctor and scientist himself, he should at least discuss the biochemistry of it with John Majnarich, Ph.D., who, as I said, is the biochemist who made the vaccine for Dr. Virginia's clinic, and who is the co-holder of the patent. Rolph did, and eventually consented to send in his urine sample. At the end of July Rolph received his vaccines, stopped his chemotherapy, and started on the vaccine protocol.

The vaccines come in three separate bottles, in concentrations of 10 million, 100 million, and 1 billion parts per million. Syringes and needles come with the vaccines. The needles are 28 gauge—no pain whatsoever! Alternatively, the vaccines can be taken sublingually. The patient simply squirts the withdrawn vaccine into a teaspoon, places the liquid under the tongue, and holds it there for 10 minutes. Complete comprehensive instructions are foolproof. The regimen calls for two doses per week; each bottle provides a ten-week regimen.

In early November 2012, Rolph called from a skiing vacation to tell me his latest blood test was absolutely normal! Not only that, but his oncologist actually told him the blood results didn't indicate he was sick with *anything,* much less leukemia. (To my great consternation, Rolph still hasn't told the oncologist about the Livingston vaccine, claiming he doesn't want her "negative vibes" to undermine his euphoria.)

Richard's Story

Another friend of a friend, Richard Lane, now seventy-three, gave me permission to use his real name and I asked him to describe in his own words his battle with an extremely rare cancer. This was his reply.

I was born in 1940 and was raised on a farm in western Minnesota. During summers, heaving 75-pound hay bales around made me fairly strong and muscular. I was a good student and an accomplished athlete. I received advanced degrees in engineering and business from the University of Minnesota. Immediately after graduation I was hired by Honeywell, Inc., as a design engineer, and rose to become general manager of a semiconductor operation in Denver. I retired from Honeywell in 1999, at age fifty-nine, after thirty-seven years of service.

During my life, I remained physically fit, jogging regularly, and doing weight training since my mid-twenties. I never smoked cigarettes, but I did enjoy daily cigars until I was in my mid-fifties. I consumed two or three glasses of wine a day, but otherwise ate a relatively healthy diet.

Late in 2001, I began to feel lethargic and to show signs of jaundice. I consulted with a doctor who immediately referred me to undergo an endoscopy procedure (a fiberoptic camera inserted down your throat to examine the stomach and duodenum areas). A tissue sample was taken of my ampulla of Vater and biopsied. (The ampulla is a nipple-like projection into the duodenum, the first portion of the intestine; it is at the confluence of the bile and pancreatic ducts, with an opening that permits secreted digestive fluids to be injected into the duodenum.) The biopsy-identified cancer had infected the ampulla and this was restricting these digestive fluids from entering the duodenum. Ampullary cancer (technically, adenocarcinoma of the ampulla of Vater) is quite rare—on the order of 3,000 cases worldwide annually. The cause is unknown. I felt I had encountered lottery-type odds: 3,000 cases in a worldwide population of 6,000,000,000—that's 1 in 2,000,000—only I had lost the lottery. My first reaction was shock, as I truly believed I had led a relatively healthy lifestyle. I immediately thought my life would soon be over.

A surgeon at a hospital in Minneapolis told my wife, Karen, and I that the requisite treatment for ampullary cancer was a Whipple surgery. A procedure in which the ampulla, parts of the bile and pancreatic ducts, part of the pancreas, the gall bladder, the duodenum, and some surrounding lymph nodes are removed. I then expressed an interest in getting a second opinion. Fortunately, we live in a state with first-rate health-care options.

I said I wished to go to Mayo Clinic Cancer Center in Rochester, where I had previous experience. The Minneapolis surgeon was sympathetic, and said he had studied under one of the world's foremost Whipple surgeons at the Mayo Clinic. An appointment was arranged, and within a week I visited him. I discovered he dealt almost exclusively with Whipple procedures, and had an entire hospital floor dedicated to his Whipple patients with teams of pre-op, operation procedures, and rehab specialists.

Within two weeks, I had the Whipple procedure. It's terribly painful the first few days after the surgery, as your entire abdominal area is exceedingly sore. After all, you've been gutted like a fish on your front side, had numerous parts removed, re-plumbed, and closed back up. But the secret to recovery, I was told, was to force myself up from bed and begin walking. I did this on day two—painful to say the least. Since I was in reasonably good physical shape prior to the operation, I recovered quite quickly and was released in seven days. (In the 1970s, 15 percent of patients died during or shortly after surgery. It's now less than 1 percent. However, the survival rate after five years is still only 20–30 percent.) Also, an ancillary effect of a Whipple is an increased tendency to develop diabetes—a result of removing part of the pancreas.

Post-op, the surgeon felt quite confident he had eliminated all the cancerous cells. He had removed organs, or parts of organs, and ducting in the vicinity of the ampulla, and had biopsied the nearby lymph nodes. Tests were negative for cancerous cells.

Following the Whipple procedure, the Mayo medical staff conferred about any need for additional treatments. The consensus was that chemotherapy was not required, and that radiation would likely do more harm than good. I convalesced at home over the next several months, making sure I did a lot of walking. After six months, I don't recall any side effects at all.

It was recommended that I see an oncologist at the Mayo Clinic every three months to monitor my post-op progress, and he ordered regular positron emission tomography (PET) scans of my abdominal area, as well as blood chemistry tests. After five years, he concluded that, based on experience in the medical community, no cancer was evidenced and that I could stop his periodic exams. Definitely, an upper for Karen and me.

But in 2008, I began to experience middle back pains. I attempted to counter the pain with ibuprofen-type medications, but to no avail. Suspecting that this was more serious than a simple back pain that would go away with time, I returned to the Mayo Clinic. Tests revealed that indeed, cancerous tumors on my lymph nodes were growing in my abdomen. One of these tumors was exerting pressure on my central nervous system and causing the back pain. According to the oncologist, I now had stage IV (late-stage) metastatic ampullary cancer, indicating the original ampullary cancer had remained dormant for about seven years but now was again active. The recommended treatment was chemotherapy.

Over the next year, I traveled to the Mayo Clinic every three weeks (200 miles round trip) to receive a chemo infusion of the drug gemcitabine (Gemzar). I also took a daily oral pill called capecitabine (Xeloda) for two of the three weeks. (Ampullary cancer is so rare that drug companies and researchers don't have enough incentive to develop specific drugs for it. Instead chemo drugs used in the treatment of pancreatic cancer are used as a proxy, since oncologists apparently regard the two forms of cancer as first cousins.) The infusion took about two hours to administer. Over time, PET scans showed a reduction in the size of my tumors.

Side effects of this chemo include, among other things, lower white and red blood cell counts, and lower platelet counts. The platelet issue is the oncologist's major concern, as platelets are required to clot blood after an injury. If the platelet count is too low, chemo treatment cannot be administered. So the routine for me was to drive the two hours to the Mayo Clinic, have a blood draw, wait for 30 minutes for its analysis, and if the platelet count was above a minimum threshold, get the infusion treatment. Occasionally, however, the platelet count was below the minimum threshold, in which case I had to forego chemo and wait for my platelet count to increase (typically, one to two weeks). Whenever I failed the platelet test, the total time consumed was at least half a day, including drive time and blood analysis. I, therefore, decided to transfer my chemo treatment to the University of Minnesota Physicians Group in Minneapolis, close to my home and only a 30-minute trip.

At the university I was fortunate to be assigned to one of their leading oncologists, who continued the Gemzar/Xeloda regimen of treatments prescribed by the Mayo Clinic for two more years, with regular monitoring of my blood chemistry and PET scans every three months. At this time (2010), my oncologist concluded that the Gemzar/Xeloda drugs had stopped being effective, as the PET scans showed growth of the abdominal lymph nodes again. Apparently, the cancerous cells had "learned" about the Gemzar/Xeloda attacks, and mutated to evade the drug's effectiveness.

At this time the oncologist referenced a research program sponsored by the pharmaceutical company Novartis that had a promising new experimental drug and needed patients like myself. Six patients at the university, plus others at similar institutions around the country, were selected and treatments began using this experimental drug. The side effects were horrendous for me (ear and sinus infections, etc.) and for the others, and PET scans showed no beneficial effect. The study was summarily discontinued.

An interesting side issue that I observed during my chemo treatments was the strong influence of insurance companies in deciding which drugs could be used by oncologists. Since I had an infrequent, peripheral type of cancer (ampullary), oncologists were required to get pre-approval for a forthcoming treatment. More than once, my insurance company rejected the use of a drug recommended by my oncologist, which normally was a drug prescribed for pancreatic cancers. The total time consumed by my oncologist to get written approval was typically two weeks. The oncologist argued that his decision was based upon the similarities to pancreatic cancer. (It seemed so ironic that a trained, experienced oncologist had to negotiate with an insurance company bureaucrat to obtain approval.)

I recall several times that, in my discussions with the oncologist, he was amazed that I was still doing reasonably well in my life. He suggested that his expectation was that I should have been dead two to three years earlier, as I had stage-IV cancer. But a saving grace was that I had slow-growing tumors which responded well to chemo, and that I was in reasonably good physical shape otherwise.

He then had another drug in his tool kit called doxorubicin (Adriamycin). In 2011, I began getting infusions, which lasted about a year. In April 2012, I apparently blacked out while driving and hit a mailbox before stopping. Karen immediately took me to the hospital where it was determined that I had excessive amounts of ammonia in my blood. (My understanding is that the healthy liver normally removes ammonia from the bloodstream, which is then eliminated from the body in your excrement. My liver system was clearly not working properly.)

Now I was at a crossroad. I was advised that continuing chemo treatments would likely cause further damage to my liver, and that the benefits were minimal. Besides, the oncologist had expended most every drug from his arsenal that could possibly help me. I had now been butchered and poisoned for close to twelve years, and I was thankful for prolonging my life that long. I had since had two wonderful grandchildren born and was thankful I at least had an opportunity to observe these bright kids grow ever older. My interpretation of the oncologist's advice was to "let nature take its course." Of course, that meant only one thing: the end was near. It was even clearer when he began discussing hospice care. I accepted this decision, as I believed he and the rest of the medical community had done as much as they could to prolong a reasonably good quality of life for me. My last chemo infusion was in April 2012.

I now began what I describe as a wind-down process for my life. I had always wanted to take an extended trip West on Amtrak. In September, Karen and I embarked on a month-long trip to Seattle, Portland, San Francisco, and Denver. On our visit to San Francisco, we met up with a high school classmate of Karen's living in Mill Valley. Her husband is a physician who had heard about my predicament and, over dinner, he mentioned he had a friend, Edmond G. Addeo, who was working on a book about the work of Dr. Virginia Livingston-Wheeler, who had discovered a cancer-causing microbe and had developed a vaccine to stimulate the immune system against it. He thought this information might be of interest to my situation and recommended we look into it and act accordingly.

Upon returning home in October, I did not feel motivated to contact Mr. Addeo about his book. Thankfully, Karen did and and was impressed with the Livingston-Wheeler message. Basically, Dr. Livingston-Wheeler believed that cancer was a bacterial (rather than a viral) infection which a person's autoimmune system was not responding adequately to, and that a vaccine and dietary changes could enhance the body's own ability to combat the cancer. This was a book obviously relevant to my battle with cancer. I had lost hope for a cure, given that some of the best medical experts in the world had capitulated on my situation.

As 2012 was coming to a close, I began feeling differently. I slept a lot and my head felt spacey. I paid increasingly little attention to conversations around me, and I could recognize that my ability to listen and respond was slowing down. I had to struggle to remember names, even people I once knew well. Whereas most of my life I had been somewhat quick-witted, I was now out of that mode. I began to walk slower, and my balance was thrown off. Physically, my muscle tone had declined markedly. My arms, thighs, chest, and buttocks were those of a ninety-year-old. My face was ashen. Friends and acquaintances saw all this, but were too polite to mention it around me.

By the New Year, Karen went into action. She had contacted the supplier of Dr. Livingston-Wheeler's immune vaccine. Also, we showed the book to my oncologist, who admitted that research work was ongoing in the field of vaccines to treat cancer but that nothing conclusive had come to fruition. However, he stated he had no objection to our pursuing the vaccine treatment method so long as it didn't break us financially. His exact comment at the end was, "What have you got to lose?"

In late January I began injecting myself twice weekly with the vaccine using a small, painless syringe, and taking abscisic acid tablets [more on this potent cancer-fighting plant hormone later]. I recalled repeating to myself: "What have I got to lose?"

In late March I sent a urine sample to the supplier for analysis and was told it showed a marked decrease in the cancer marker human chorionic gonadotropin (HCG), a hormone produced by certain cancer cells. "The treatment is working as it's supposed to," the biochemist stated, "the tumors are shrinking." A recent blood test by my oncologist revealed that the cancer blood marker carcinoembryonic antigen (CEA), a protein in the blood, had also decreased markedly in the last three months.

In addition, I am now on a much more stringent diet than at any time in my life. I try to avoid foods and substances that can weaken my immune system. This means I consume no sugar, no high-fructose corn syrup, no artificial sweeteners, no pork, and no alcohol. I also use no deodorants with parabens (a type of preservative), take no flu shots, and had my dental amalgam fillings removed.

I have now resumed working out physically, using a treadmill and weights. My muscle tone has improved considerably. My spaciness has largely disappeared and my balance is back. My skin color has returned to normal. I often now hear from people I previously had regular contact with about how healthy I look.

Acquaintances frequently ask what's in this vaccine I inject and how do I know it's safe. My response is that for four years, I took chemo drugs and hadn't the slightest idea what was in them. I only knew the Food and Drug Administration (FDA) had approved them, mostly for safety I expect, and that they were very expensive. One of the chemo drugs employed had a list price of $22,000. Of course, the negotiated price for insurance purposes was about 10 percent of this, or $2,200. So using this vaccine was no scarier for me than using chemo drugs, and a lot cheaper. I mostly relied upon previous users' experiences and could not comprehend a sinister motive to provide me with a drug that was unsafe.

But another way to view this is that the really serious cancers like liver or pancreatic cancer have high fatality rates. For pancreatic cancer, only 20 percent of infected patients live beyond one year. For late-stage cancer patients like myself, half will die in two to six months. Similarly, the expected survival time for stage-IV liver cancer is three to six months. Thus, administering chemotherapy to these patients is likely to prolong life only for a short time. Patients likely spend a lot of resources for a short reprieve on life expectancy, and with a decreased quality of life.

At this time, I certainly can't conclude that I've conquered cancer. I may still pass early. But at least I've been given a gift to live a bit longer with a relatively healthy lifestyle. If the reader would like to follow up with me and learn more, please contact me through the publisher.

Janice's Story

Janice M. is sixty-seven and lives in Florida. Her primary care physician, a medical doctor who practices integrative medicine, called her into her office in May 2012 after finding through routine blood work an elevated white blood cell count. The doctor said she was concerned with the way Janice's blood sample looked and she told her that she suspected either lymphoma (cancer of the lymph system) or leukemia. At this point she referred her to an oncologist. The oncologist diagnosed her with CLL, the same condition as my friend Rolph.

The oncologist recommended chemotherapy at the point when her white blood cell doubled. As her white blood cells continued to rise and Janice was unwilling to undergo chemotherapy, she consulted with an alternative doctor in February 2013. She started his protocol in March 2013, which included intravenous ozone therapy and ozone enemas; vitamins C, K, B_{12}; and intravenous glutathione therapy; as well as hyperbaric chamber therapy. Part of her protocol was also taking no less than 200 supplements daily, 24 hours around the clock. When by coincidence, a close friend who is a holistic healer happened to call, Janice told her about her supplement regimen, and the friend told her it was "ludicrous" and "beyond madness" to take so many supplements, that her body didn't even know how to process such amounts. In late June, Janice stopped all supplements and re-assessed her options.

In early May, a friend told her about the Livingston vaccine still being available and she started on the protocol. At that time her urine marker was 36 nanograms (ng) of HCG per milliliter (mL). When Janice sent her urine sample to the lab two months later, in July, to order her maintenance bottles, her marker had come down to 26 ng of HCG per mL, and by the end of July her marker was down to 16 ng of HCG per mL.

When I spoke with Janice just before this book went to press, she was feeling great and her condition was greatly improved. Her white blood cell count was still down dramatically and she had abundant energy and felt completely normal.

Wilson's Story

Just before this book went to press I received a call from a man who had a history of cancer and had visited the Livingston-Wheeler Clinic in San Diego. He was very excited about the continued existence of the Livingston immune vaccine. His story is among the most interesting of all.

Thirty years ago, Wilson Parasiuk, a Canadian, was diagnosed with a malignant melanoma under his left thumbnail. Malignant melanoma is an aggressive type of skin cancer that can spread rapidly. The tumor was deeply imbedded within the flesh and around the blood vessels and bones. Furthermore, the tumor had been cut through when the general practitioner tried to take a sample for a biopsy. The prognosis for Wilson was grim. He was told that a significant amputation was to be pursued (possibly the hand, the forearm, or the entire arm). Hopefully the surgery would slow down the melanoma as there was no chemotherapy or radiation procedures for advanced, deeply imbedded melanoma tumors. At the same time Wilson's wife was quietly told that the odds were that her husband would likely die in as little as three months so the family should "organize its affairs" accordingly.

Wilson insisted that only the left thumb be amputated. This was done in Winnipeg, but then he was told that the normal follow-up procedure would be to remove his lymph nodes under his arms and in his groin area. He was told that the removal of these lymph nodes would likely have significant side effects. To Wilson, this approach seemed totally illogical, since his life expectancy was so short.

Wilson sought out a second opinion. He visited a world-famous cancer treatment center in New York City. There, it was confirmed that he had an advanced case of melanoma. The treatment center recommended amputating Wilson's whole arm and that, as a matter of policy, he would then have his lymph nodes removed. Wilson thought this seemed just as illogical as the program that was proposed to him in Winnipeg. He asked about alternatives like diet and visualization and was curtly told that they did not believe in quackery. In short, the traditionalists had nothing to offer and he was left on his own with his family to "organize his affairs."

Wilson and his extended family then took a winter vacation in January 1984, to Palm Springs, California, as a potential last gathering of the extended Parasiuk family. While in Palm Springs, Wilson came across the book I wrote with Dr. Virginia Livingston-Wheeler, *The Conquest of Cancer: Vaccines and Diet.* Wilson and his wife immediately went to the Livingston-Wheeler Clinic in nearby San Diego. There, he undertook the full Livingston treatment protocol of vaccines, diet, antibiotics, and other modalities (discussed in Chapter 2), The expected life expectancy of three months lapsed into six months, then one year, then two, three, and four years as he continued the treatment. After five years, Wilson stopped further treatment. The melanoma was gone and he had no related recurrence.

Wilson told people who asked him about his experience with melanoma cancer and his treatment to look into the published works of Dr. Livingston-Wheeler and decide for themselves what they should do. Unfortunately, most people did not go to the clinic, preferring to stay solely with the advice of their traditionalist doctors. Wilson told these people, many of whom had more illustrious academic credentials than their doctors, that they should be "subjects, not objects" in exploring their treatment alternatives. "Unfortunately, these people slavishly followed their doctors' advice and, ultimately, died," Wilson says. "The few independent thinkers that did go to the Livingston-Wheeler Clinic either survived or had their quality of life greatly improved as their condition progressed. Not all the people who went to the clinic with advanced cancer lived. However, no person I ever met who went to the clinic ever had misgivings about having gone."

In due course, Wilson heard that Dr. Virginia had died and that her clinic had been closed. Life went on. Then, in 2009, he was diagnosed with a very aggressive prostate cancer and without recourse to the Livingston immunity vaccine he had prostate cancer surgery. Indeed, at that time, Wilson reflected that Dr. Virginia had never been against surgery to remove a cancer mass. He was told by his surgeon, as have been so many others with cancer, that they had "got it all." Unfortunately, within a few years Wilson's prostate-specific antigen (PSA) levels began to ominously rise. (PSA is a protein produced by the prostate cells; high levels may indicate the presence of prostate cancer.) He was told that if the rise in PSA levels continued various treatments like hormonal therapy and other "more intrusive" treatments might be required.

Parasiuk was ultimately referred by one medical doctor to Dr. Majnarich's laboratory in Redmond. He visited the lab, conferred with Dr. Majnarich, and started on the vaccine protocol. Currently, his PSA levels have leveled off and have begun to decline.

Wilson has become an energetic and vocal supporter of the concept of cancer being an immunological disease in general and of the immune vaccine in particular. He is disturbed that so much of what Dr. Virginia and others had pioneered and championed has languished under attack from the medical and pharmaceutical establishment, especially since her death. Wilson believes that Dr. Virginia's approach and demonstrated successes warrant present day re-examination, application, and availability to interested people who seek alternatives for their care and treatment.

Imagine my surprise when he told me that he was a former minister of health in the government of Manitoba, Canada!

Remarkable Stories

"I can't see why the medical profession keeps skirting around the evidence," Dr. Majnarich says. "Maybe in a year or so they'll pick up on the microbial causes of cancer. They certainly must be getting close, because related studies reported in reputable journals are piling higher every month."

When I referred to some of these case histories as "miracles," Dr. Majnarich said, "They're *not* miracles! The vaccine is doing exactly what it's *supposed* to do!"

As I've mentioned, one serious problem I've had all too frequently in my research is that doctors who are using the Livingston vaccine protocol to boost immunity are not willing to come out of the closet and admit it in public. Understandably, they are afraid of losing their license—which happens when docs deviate from surgery, chemotherapy, and radiation. (Called "cut, poison, and burn" in some circles.)

Unfortunately, the Health Insurance Portability and Accountability Act (HIPAA) of 1996 prevents agencies from giving me the names of any of those physicians. And of those I managed to identify by other means and then interviewed, all refused to let me use their names. One threatened to sue me if I did. An integrative clinic in Santa Rosa, California, never returned my calls or answered my emails, and when I actually visited them and knocked on their front door, I was told that the doctor in charge was "traveling." Richard Lane's oncologist never answered emails or returned calls. To be fair, docs can't discuss patients' treatments without written permission—but he could have at least told me that. Besides, Richard gave him permission to talk to me. And I know for certain that he ordered a copy of the book—Richard actually saw him order it from Amazon. Whether he read it or not is another story.

Yet, exciting as these patient reports are, I think it would be help-ful to start at the beginning of my journey into writing about this remarkable woman.

2

A Glutton for Punishment?

About thirty years ago I approached a palatial seaside home in La Jolla, California, and knocked on the front door of the most remarkable woman I have ever met. The event would change my life in dramatic ways, because I had been invited to collaborate with this distinguished woman on a book that would bring her story to the American people. As I knocked, I had grave misgivings: this woman claimed she had the cure for cancer and I wanted nothing whatsoever to do with quacks.

Amid continual brickbats and derision from the medical establishment, Virginia Livingston-Wheeler, M.D., loudly and vociferously claimed she had discovered a microbe that was the cause of cancer, and that she could cure the disease with a combination of immune-boosting vaccinations and a vitamin-rich dietary regimen. What's more, she asserted that she had been treating thousands of patients at her immunotherapy clinic in San Diego with a 90 percent cure rate (her critics wished her to use the term "remission"), and that she would quite willingly turn over their medical charts and all her internal records to any qualified individuals, professional agencies, or investigative bodies who wanted to examine her work for themselves.

Quite a challenge. Would a quack be so forthcoming with her records when mainstream medicine had already come out against her? If she were an avaricious charlatan, would she risk everything by inviting the scrutiny of peers known to be predisposed to condemn her? And would a highly qualified medical doctor with impeccable educational and experiential credentials, who was already accused of opportunism and profiteering from the sick and desperate, publicly invite her critics to prove her wrong?

Yet no one appeared at her clinic to call her bluff. The American Cancer Society (ACS) was merciless in its incessant dismissal of her theories, yet never showed up to examine her practices. The National Cancer Institute (NCI) didn't come. The U.S. Centers for Disease Control and Prevention (CDC) didn't come. The Federal Drug Administration (FDA) didn't come. The American Medical Association (AMA) didn't come. No one came to peer into her microscopes, or to interview her patients, or to analyze her vaccines.

In fact, not until 1991 did a "Special Article" appear in the prestigious *New England Journal of Medicine*, which "vigorously debated" the value of cancer treatments of "unproved efficacy." Entitled "Survival and Quality of Life Among Patients Receiving Unproven as Compared with Conventional Cancer Therapy," the article reported on a study undertaken at the University of Pennsylvania and funded by the National Institutes of Health (NIH), in which 78 patients at Pennsylvania Hospital were compared with 78 patients of the Livingston-Wheeler Medical Clinic. To make a long story short, the study concluded that Dr. Virginia's patients fared no better or worse than conventional therapy patients. The clinic's proponents claim the article failed to point out that most of Dr. Virginia's patients had been declared "terminal" by the time they first presented at the clinic. Alas, Dr. Virginia died shortly after the completion of the study, and never had the chance to comment officially on the study's methodology, hypotheses, and conclusions.

My Introduction to Dr. Virginia by Happenstance

Dr. Virginia had been a well-known and indefatigable researcher into the bacteriology and epidemiology of cancer for many years. Not being a medical professional myself, I first ran across her name in 1972 when, after a near-death episode of pneumonia combined with the news that my father had bladder cancer, I decided to find out all I could about optimum health in general and cancer specifically.

My research got a kick-start with Dr. Linus Pauling's now celebrated pronouncements about ascorbic acid's immune-boosting properties. As I read his work and eventually met him for an extensive interview, it seemed peculiar that this brilliant man, who had twice won a Nobel Prize—one for Chemistry (1954), the other for Peace (1962)—was being chastised and downright scorned by his colleagues. The medical establishment came out against him, vilified his claims that high doses of ascorbic acid—vitamin C—could palliate, if not prevent, the common cold. Dr. Pauling's thesis was that vitamin C is an essential ingredient that helps our cells carry on a defensive immune process called "phagocytosis," in which the cell envelops and digests harmful foreign bodies. Dr. Pauling's studies showed that higher levels of vitamin C than we normally have in our bodies could ward off the viruses that give us colds and infections. But the medical community scoffed and generally dismissed him as an eccentric. It wasn't until the '80s that mainstream doctors started accepting his theory, because it started to make sense as new studies began to confirm it.

Before Dr. Pauling's sensational thesis, a biochemist named Dr. Irwin Stone theorized that, by reason of a genetic "accident" millions of years ago, we human beings lost our ability to synthesize a certain enzyme required in the production of ascorbic acid in the body. Hence, we started taking in ascorbic acid exogenously (from outside sources) by eating leaves, plants, and roots, until today we are one of the few mammals on earth that doesn't manufacture its own ascorbic acid. Therefore, Dr. Stone postulated, we are all walking around with what he called "chronic subclinical scurvy," or CSS, that is only palliated by our intake of ascorbic acid-bearing foods.

Dr. Pauling, building on classic immune-system theory, took Dr. Stone's thesis one step further and formulated his vitamin C versus the common cold theory. Many scientists (including Dr. Virginia, as we'll see) have since considered the proposition that if a little extra vitamin C can boost our immunity to prevent colds and scurvy, then perhaps regular doses of vitamin C could help our bodies ward off other diseases as well—simply by maintaining a stronger immune system and hence a higher level of health in general.

Dr. Pauling then extended his research into cancer, and with Scottish physician Ewan Cameron, published several papers proposing that ascorbic acid had palliative effects on cancer patients, and in fact could be an effective immune-boosting element in cancer therapy.

It is both amusing and aggravating now to recall that when I mentioned the possibility of high doses of ascorbic acid to my father's doctor, he scoffed and said he was afraid my father would develop kidney stones. When I reminded him that my father was dying of cancer and kidney stones were the least of our worries, he grudgingly put my father on 50 milligrams (mg) of vitamin C per day. *Fifty* mg! And Dr. Pauling was recommending 10,000 mg per day, and several other physicians were recommending between 40,000 and 50,000 mg per day just for the sniffles!

As Dr. Pauling's writings guided my reading from the common cold to cancer, I began to notice something else peculiar. In every paper and study I ran across that had something positive or promising to say about a cancer treatment (i.e., a remission or a diminution in size of a tumor), there were always two things mentioned: 1) vitamin A, or an analog thereof, and 2) the name Dr. Virginia Livingston.

My Introduction to Dr. Virginia Through Other Physicians

In the late 1970s I met two physicians who were in the vanguard of supporting Dr. Virginia's work and who were not afraid to practice what she preached. One was Rex E. Wiederanders, M.D., a prominent Midwestern surgeon and the author of more than twenty professional articles. I referred some of my research to him in order to confirm medical accuracy and sound scientific methods. When I asked him about this Dr. Virginia Livingston I had been reading about, he wrote, "After twenty years of surgical practice and having seen innumerable patients die the anguished death of cancer, and seeing no significant decrease in that number from the standard treatment modalities, I feel [Dr. Virginia's] method of immunotherapy is the most enlightened, the most promising, and the one that should be pursued with enthusiasm. The more quickly we follow this great pioneer's lead, the more lives will be saved."

The second physician I met was Richard A. Kunin, M.D., who had lectured and written extensively on the subject of nutrition and health, and who was then a founder and president of the Orthomolecular Medical Society, an organization of medical doctors who embraced nutritional and some other alternative therapies in their respective practices. His opinion: "Dr. Virginia Livingston-Wheeler [she had then remarried to Owen Wheeler, M.D.] has succeeded in devising a scientifically rational program for the prevention and treatment of cancer, incorporating a scientific program of vaccines and diet to successfully support the immune system in the destruction of cancer cells. This isn't mere theory—the conquest of cancer is now at hand."

My Introduction to Dr. Virginia Through Her Work

Finally, because of my association with Dr. Kunin, I happened to be at an Orthomolecular Medical Society meeting in January 1980, in San Francisco, at which hundreds of physicians were in attendance. I listened to Dr. Virginia present a paper on the immunotherapy program at her clinic. With the aid of her husband Owen Webster

Wheeler, M.D., she presented a wealth of scientific research data with slides and charts, microphotographs, patient histories, and a description of her early work with laboratory animals. A wealth of data was displayed as she explained her discovery of the cancer-causing microbe and her successful treatment program, which emphasized the strengthening of her patients' immune systems.

Dr. Virginia described a treatment program that consisted of giving patients:

- Antitubercular vaccines (bacillus Calmette-Guerin, or BCG, essentially a TB shot) to boost immune response.

- Autogenous vaccines (sometimes referred to autologous vaccines) prepared from the patient's own tumor, that is, from a culture of the patient's infectious microbe.

- Antibiotics (since she claimed cancer was an infectious disease).

- High doses of vitamins A, C, and E, and essential minerals.

- An immunity-boosting diet consisting of a largely vegetarian whole-foods diet, with a major emphasis on the inclusion of cruciferous vegetables such as broccoli, cauliflower, Brussels sprouts, cabbage, and kale, and the avoidance of "cancer-promoting foods," like refined sugars, processed foods, poultry (more on this later), as well as alcohol, coffee, and cigarettes.

- A little-known plant hormone and vitamin-A derivative called abscisic acid that she found to be a particularly strong anticancer agent (to learn more, see "Vitamin A and Abscisic Acid," page 23).

Dr. Virginia concluded her presentation by reporting that, although her treatment program could still be expanded, she was achieving an improvement rate among her patients in excess of 90 percent. The austere medical audience gave her a ten-minute standing ovation. It was very impressive.

I spent the next two years becoming more familiar with ortho-molecular medicine in general and Dr. Virginia's work in particular. I learned that her bacteriology work had been published in respected journals; that while a professor of microbiology at Rutgers University and then as a researcher at Memorial Sloan-Kettering Cancer Center, her work had been applauded at major medical meetings from Rome to Paris to New York; and that she was listed in *Who's Who in Science and Medicine.*

VITAMIN A AND ABSCISIC ACID

Vitamin A is commonly known as the anti-infective vitamin, because it is required for normal functioning of the immune system. Dr. Virginia recommended a lot of vitamin A and vitamin A analogs (derivatives or variants of the real vitamin) in her immunotherapy program.

One of these vitamin A analogs known as abscisic acid is a plant hormone that mainly acts to inhibit growth, promote dormancy, and help plants and deciduous trees tolerate stressful conditions such as the onset of winter. In the body, Dr. Virginia discovered that abscisic acid could fortify the body's defense mechanisms and suppress susceptibility to infection by cancer-causing microbes. She found it to be abundant in young, flowering broccoli (specifically, sprouts to the age of eight days), in other cruciferous vegetables, and in certain fruits like the apricot. She postulated that abscisic acid was the most potent chemoprotector in our food. (This substance was later developed by Dr. John Majnarich, the biochemist who made the vaccine for Dr. Virginia's clinic, into a powerful concentrated pill, called CIS-14, which his lab also supplies to cancer patients.)

Since then, a lot of research studies have shown that foods high in vitamin A are strong chemoprotectors against cancer. For more on broccoli sprouts, tomatoes, and other powerful vitamin-A rich anticancer foods, read on.

My Introduction to Dr. Virginia Herself

In June of 1982, I met Bill Gladstone, a literary agent who was friendly with Dr. Virginia, and who was searching for a seasoned science writer to help bring her story to the American public. Because my friendships with Drs. Wiederanders and Kunin had resulted in two scientific books co-written with each, as well as seven other books published by mainstream New York houses, Bill was familiar with my work. (See his foreword for more on these events.) He asked if I'd heard of her. I gave him chapter and verse, and he asked if I'd be interested in collaborating with her on a book through which she wanted to bring her complex and dramatic medical story to the general reader. Despite what I'd read and heard, at first I was reluctant. I didn't want to risk a budding writing career by affiliating myself with a kook—someone who would ultimately be shown to be using smoke and mirrors to produce her so-called cures.

I finally told Bill that I'd be willing to meet with Dr. Virginia, visit her clinic and tour the facilities, and personally interview a random sampling of her patients. This I was allowed to do, and more. Not only did I look through her microscopes, speak with her patients, and thoroughly study her published papers (under the tutelage of a biochemist friend), but also—carefully avoiding her known detractors with their negative agendas—I talked with several impartial scientists and medical doctors. The verdict from almost all of them was on the order of, "I don't know why no one's taken the time to replicate her work, because she hasn't stepped out of any boundaries of medicine, but what she's doing certainly *could* be valid."

Armed with such carefully worded evaluations and opinions couched in conditional phrasings, I agreed to work with Dr. Virginia. I soon found myself engrossed in what I came to consider one of the most exciting possibilities of the twentieth century. After many weeks spent in her clinic, after hundreds of hours staying with her and Dr. Wheeler at their home in La Jolla, and after interviewing hundreds of patients and reviewing hundreds of medical charts, I became convinced—and still am—that some day her work will be deemed as important as that of Louis Pasteur, Marie Curie, and Jonas Salk/Albert Sabin.

Validation, Slowly but Surely

After Dr. Virginia's death, certain studies began appearing in medical journals that approached confirmation of her work, but never quite attributed any research findings to her. One study, reported in the January 2008 issue of the *Journal of Urology*, presented a remarkable remission rate among nineteen women with uterine cancer after having been treated with BCG vaccines. Oncologists soon after began treating bladder cancer with BCG. Researchers at Memorial Sloan-Kettering Cancer Center, the nation's oldest and largest research and hospital complex devoted exclusively to cancer, have become leaders in the study of autogenous vaccines in the treatment of cancers of the bladder, blood, breast, prostate, and skin. A major report revealed that lycopenes (contained in abundance in vitamin A-rich vegetables, especially tomatoes and fruits) had strong immune-boosting properties and could be potent anticancer nutrients (page 63). And the National Academy of Sciences (NAS), a research organization that advises the federal government and the public on scientific and technical matters, issued a report in its September 1997 *Proceedings* that concluded unequivocally that the sprouts of young broccoli were powerful anticancer agents (see page 26).

Remember Linus Pauling, a Nobel Laureate ridiculed for his theory about vitamin C and the common cold (and cancer). Remember Louis Pasteur, hooted off the stage in Paris when he presented his "germ" theory. Remember Ignaz Philip Semmelweis, driven out of Vienna for insisting that students and physicians wash their hands after autopsies and before delivering babies. These great figures went from living pariahs to dead pioneers when their "radical" theories were found to be valid.

News Update:
Researchers Say Broccoli Fights Cancer

A headline in the September 17, 1997, *San Francisco Chronicle* caught my eye: "Broccoli Sprouts Called a Potent Cancer Foe." At first, I thought it was about some tabloid hawking broccoli as a "miracle cure." Eat broccoli, fight cancer—obviously another quack diet in the making. But no. The article was about a report in that month's *Proceedings of the National Academy of Sciences,* in which three scientists at the Johns Hopkins University School of Medicine, led by Paul Talalay, M.D., discovered that eating broccoli sprouts is "a powerful strategy for achieving protection against carcinogenesis."

Young broccoli sprouts, as well as other cruciferous plants like brussels sprouts, cauliflower, and kale, boost the immune system and fight against toxic agents that may lead to malignancies. A quick trip to the Internet supplied Dr. Talalay's full 14-page report. Young broccoli sprouts, as well as cruciferous vegetables like brussels sprouts have lots of isothiocyanates, sulfur-containing compounds that help give it up to 100 times the cancer-fighting power of mature broccoli.

Since the 1997 NAS paper, Dr. Talalay and his colleagues have identified an isothiocyanate, called sulforaphane, and its natural precursor, sulforaphane glucosinolate (SGS), that are thought to be key factors in many of the health benefits attributed to cruciferous vegetables. The scientists in his laboratory believe that sulforaphane inhibits enzymes, called histone deacetylases (HDACs), which are known to work against the ability of certain genes to suppress the development of tumors, and that SGS boosts the body's own antioxidant defense system, including phase 2 detoxification enzymes, which promote long-lasting antioxidant activity in the body. These Johns Hopkins University researchers found that three-day-old broccoli sprouts, in particular, contained exceptionally high concentrations of sulforaphane and SGS.

While performing their research, the scientists found that certain types of broccoli sprouts contain higher levels of the compound than others. Talalay and his group set out to determine which of the 98 varieties of broccoli seeds would guarantee a high and consistent level of SGS. After identifying the particular seed and optimal growing conditions, Talalay patented the sprout. Originally called BroccoSprouts, but since re-named Life Force Sandwich Blend, these powerful broccoli sprouts are now available in grocery stores throughout the country. (Dr. Talalay and Johns Hopkins have divested themselves from any financial interest in the product and receive no profit whatsoever from its sale.)

In addition to Dr. Talalay's work, there are at least two-dozen clinical studies now being conducted on the chemoprotective qualities of young broccoli sprouts. One of these studies reported in the journal *Clinical Epigenetics* showed that sulforaphane also works in another way to fight cancer, through a mechanism called DNA methylation. DNA methylation is a normal process of turning off genes, and it helps control what DNA material gets read as part of genetic communication within cells. In cancer that process gets mixed up. In the paper, researcher Emily Ho states, "It appears that DNA methylation and HDAC inhibition, both of which can be influenced by sulforaphane, work in concert with each other to maintain proper cell function. They sort of work as partners and talk to each other."

In 2010, Yanyan Li and researchers from the University of Michigan Comprehensive Cancer Center published a study in the journal *Clinical Cancer Research* showing that sulforaphane was able to kill breast cancer stem cells in mice and in lab cultures, and also prevented new tumor cells from growing.

And finally, at the Lombardi Comprehensive Cancer Center at Georgetown University, researchers reported that isothiocyanates induce apoptosis (programmed cell self-destruction) in cancer cells. In a paper published in the *Journal of Medicinal Chemistry* in 2011, the team demonstrated that certain naturally occurring isothiocyanates selectively deplete a mutant gene called p53. Mutated p53 is implicated in about half of all human cancers. Proteins coded by this gene help keep cancer from starting to grow. But when the p53 gene is mutated, the report said, that protection is gone.

Was there a vitamin A connection (discussed in the previous inset) to the NAS study?

"Definitely not," Dr. Talalay said, a bit defensively. He would say only that "raising detoxification enzymes is a good anticancer defense," and that eating lots of fruits and vegetables daily will give a person all the essential nutrients to maintain high immunity."

However, based on all the evidence, albeit circumstantial, the urge to make the connection is almost irresistible. Are the isothiocyanates in the NAS study chemically related to the apricot pit cyanides (now known to be high in abscisic acid) purported to have tumor-resistant qualities as suggested by the eminent German biochemist Hans Krebs, who won the Nobel Prize for Medicine in 1953?

One of the treatment modalities that earned Dr. Virginia much ridicule was a strict vegetarian diet that many found too stringent to follow realistically and the administration of high doses of vitamin A (as well as C and E), for the logical reason that abscisic acid is an analog of vitamin A and Dr. Virginia postulated that abscisic acid was the most potent chemoprotector in our food.

Which brings me back to the broccoli in Dr. Talalay's NAS study. If young broccoli sprouts are high in abscisic acid, and if the broccoli sprouts in Dr. Talalay's study are extremely potent chemoprotectors, then is it mere chemical coincidence that the NAS study comes very close to corroborating Dr. Virginia's theory about abscisic acid and cancer?

In other words, is it likely there are *two* potent chemoprotectors in the same vegetable? As you'll read in other News Updates, the latest data confirms Dr. Virginia's insistence on a high cruciferous diet. Never mind her microbe theory. Never mind her BCG treatment. And granted, a high vegetable and fruit diet will give us all more of *all* nutrients. But the fact that Dr. Virginia's abscisic acid and Dr. Talalay's sulforaphane are both powerful chemoprotectors in the same plant is major evidence that *that* part of her theory can take its place among several others as being accurate.

So where are we today?

Dr. Virginia was criticized for using BCG to boost the immune systems of her patients. Today, BCG has been so successful in the immunotherapy treatment of bladder cancer that not only is its use the preferred treatment, but also it has been expanded in treating colon cancer, breast cancers, squamous cell cancer, leprosy, and oral cancers.

Dr. Virginia was maligned for using autogenous vaccines made from a patient's own tumor to help that patient's immune system attack and destroy a tumor. Today, autogenous vaccines are being developed by almost every major medical center and university, and at this writing the FDA has approved four vaccines for commercial use, most notably in 2010 a vaccine for the treatment of prostate cancer (page 163).

Dr. Virginia proposed that cancer was caused not by a virus, but by a bacterium that *behaved* like a virus. Today, in one of the great medical reversals of the last generation, stomach ulcers not only have been shown to be precursors of cancer but also to be caused by the bacterium *Helicobacter pylori*, which is treatable with antibiotics (page 121).

And Dr. Virginia advocated a high intake of cancer-fighting, immune-boosting nutrients such as vitamin A and its analog abscisic acid. Today, stories about vitamin A-based foods versus cancer abound. While they usually stop short of recommending vitamin A supplements, the ACS, the NCI, and some other reputable researchers now recommend that we add more cruciferous vegetables and other foods high in carotenes (vitamin A) to our diets.

Dr. Virginia never achieved the fame—or notoriety, for that matter—of such medical heroes as Pasteur, Curie, and other celebrated pioneers. But the tiny broccoli sprouts in the NAS study mentioned above were another small step in the realization that her multifaceted immunotherapy is the one program that has come closest to success after nearly a century of research.

Friends called me a glutton for punishment when I started this new book, but that NAS study and other research results pouring out of the nation's laboratories made me decide to take another look at her work and how it may be influencing the direction of cancer research today. If nothing else, I hope it shines a new light on Dr. Virginia's pioneering hypothesis and brings new hope and encouragement to cancer patients everywhere.

3

Meeting Dr. Virginia

Dr. Owen Wheeler answered the door thirty-two years ago. A short, pleasant man with sparkling eyes and a gracious, gentlemanly manner, he welcomed me and invited me to have a seat in the living room.

He suddenly shouted off to a corner of the house, "Virginia! Mr. Addeo is here!" Startled, I heard a distant voice.

"Tell him to have a seat! I'll be right up!"

I immediately became nervous, although I'm not sure why. As a young reporter in Los Angeles for the *Hollywood Citizen-News,* I had interviewed innumerable movie stars and celebrities, and in fact had hobnobbed backstage with Burt Lancaster and Elizabeth Taylor at the 1961 Academy Awards. When I was a science editor for McGraw-Hill in San Francisco, I had interviewed industrial giants and famed scientists (including Dr. Linus Pauling) from around the globe. Yet here I was becoming nervous about meeting Dr. Virginia. Maybe it was her directive to Dr. Wheeler to *tell* me to have a seat, instead of *asking* me. I was to find out soon enough that Dr. Virginia seldom *asked* people to do anything—she *told* them.

I say "living room" and "house" out of sheer habit. The place was sumptuous. I could have put the entire ground floor of my own house in her living room. The starting battery for the San Diego Padres could have warmed up in it. The entire curved front wall was glass, overlooking the cliffs of La Jolla and affording a sweeping 180-degree view of the Pacific Ocean. A grand piano stood diminutively in one corner. Dr. Virginia and Dr. Owen (as I would come to know him) would host piano concerts in the room and expect a hundred guests to attend.

Dr. Owen put me at ease immediately. He inquired about my drive down from San Francisco, about my family, and my background in general—all the while seeming genuinely interested, not just making small talk.

Some Initial Hurdles

The first problem I encountered was that Dr. Virginia didn't speak English. She spoke "Bacteriology." It became apparent as the evening wore on that I would definitely have to do a lot of translating in order to make her book comprehensible to the average person. She would use words and terms such as choriogonadotropin, *Mycobacterium avium*, and *Corynebacterium diphtheriae* with the facility and frequency that a carpenter uses the words hammer and nail. On that first night, and in the first weeks of our association, it became my routine to take copious notes, to which I would later refer and have Dr. Owen patiently explain to me what the woman was talking about.

The second problem—although short-lived—was the shock of reconciling each night what was spread before me on the dinner table and what I had been experiencing in the clinic laboratory all day. Dr. Virginia took special pains to alert her patients and everyone else to the dangers of eating chicken: most of them contained the pathogenic form of her cancer microbe, which she considered to be transmissible to human beings (more on this in Chapter 11). Yet, that first evening and on frequent occasions thereafter, I found my plate heaped with chicken! Deliciously prepared by Dr. Virginia's gourmet live-in chef, to be sure, but nevertheless—chicken! I also frequently ate eggs for breakfast, another forbidden food.

When I got up the nerve to inquire about the apparent dichotomy, it was explained to me (as if I were an infant, of course) that the food on the table before me had come from *vaccinated* chickens and was therefore free of the cancer pathogen and totally safe to eat. I also learned quickly that the clinic maintained a nearby ranch on which were raised thousands of cancer-free chickens in an ultra-hygienic environment. These chickens and their eggs were used in the clinic's cafeteria and were sold to patients and employees at cut-rate prices.

The final problem I encountered (and eventually learned to live with) was Dr. Virginia's innate Teutonic stubbornness. Here she was in her seventies, as coy and coquettish as a high school girl when she wanted to be, but frequently displaying a stubborn streak and a foot-stamping brand of obstinacy that we would call "spoiled brat" if it were applied to a two-year-old. I would later surmise that it was probably Dr. Virginia's near-dictatorial rigidity that caused her to burn her bridges behind her when she left Rutgers University and stormed out of Memorial Sloan-Kettering Cancer Center in 1953, and which perpetuated her cobra-mongoose relationship with the American Cancer Society for the rest of her years.

However, it was the case then, and has been ever since, that whenever I heard anyone who knew her mention Dr. Virginia's inflexibility, it was done so with admiration and total lack of vitriol—such was the woman's charm and sincere devotion to her Hippocratic mission. Indeed, when we tussled over the wording of the Collaborator's Note that I insisted on writing at the beginning of her book *The Conquest of Cancer,* she had cut about 3,000 words out of a 4,000-word treatise, simply because her near-total lifetime immersion in science rendered her unable to identify with certain images and reflections on my personal history. (Example: I had referred to myself in my athletic youth as a "Walter Mitty quarterback." Dr. Virginia didn't know who Walter Mitty was, and no amount of explanation on my part or random querying of friends and neighbors could convince her that it was a legitimate metaphor.)

That first evening passed quickly. Dr. Virginia appeared in a blue silk dress, modest jewelry, and moderate makeup. Her hair was stark white, coiffed. She was a short, overweight woman, but old photographs indicated her physiognomy was more of the genetically ordained "buxom" variety than the dumpy results of profligate living usually conjured by the word "overweight."

Young Virginia

We chatted into the night, I giving her some professional background and the usual details of my current personal life; she telling me bits and pieces of her early childhood. She even made the only mention I've ever heard of a secret and ill-advised marriage when she was at Vassar College to a boozing Manhattan journalist whom she called "Frank," whom she claimed had won a Pulitzer Prize, and whom she quickly divorced because of his drinking. ("It was a terrible mistake," she said, "and I was a very foolish girl.") She never mentioned him again.

Such a character doesn't appear in any of her biographical data and has never been mentioned by family or friends, but in 1922 a Frank M. O'Brien won the Pulitzer Prize for a piece called "The Unknown Soldier," published in the *New York Herald*. The date jibes, and I never heard Dr. Virginia fabricate, exaggerate, or distort a fact in the least.

Dr. Virginia recalled fondly the influence her adored father had on her life. Dr. Herman Weurthele was a respected physician in Meadville, Pennsylvania, and would frequently take his precocious daughter on his rounds with him. Dr. Virginia told me how she would ask questions and her father would explain to her everything he was doing. One can only speculate on such a picture in those pre–World War I days: a doctor visits a patient's home with a preteen female in tow, and explains to her the elements of medicine he is applying to a mystified, and maybe perturbed, patient.

If such procedures had been around in those days, she probably would have tested at a genius or near-genius level. She recalled to me how she almost had a nervous breakdown when she first encountered the concept of infinity. Even in those days, when students actually pondered scholastic concepts, it's hard to imagine a teenager becoming so distraught trying to get to the other end of parallel lines. One can only assume that she applied an inordinately precocious intelligence to her schoolwork, and especially to the subject of science. More than once she marveled those around her with what strongly appeared to be a photographic memory.

Of a typical evening, young Virginia would pester her father to read to her from his medical books, and explain to her in tedious detail the fascinating pictures and illustrations contained therein. She told me once that by the time she went off to college she thought she knew as much as any doctor, and often would be asked by her father for a diagnosis of a particular patient's condition. She would be right more often than not. Because, as I said, I found her to have a virtually photographic memory, recalling the most complicated details of medical minutiae, it was easy to believe her. But in those days the idea of a woman becoming a physician was unheard of, and so at Vassar she majored in Economics.

After she graduated, and with her turbulent secret romance behind her, she worked for a while at Macy's, but a yearning for a medical career nagged her. Eventually, she was accepted into New York University's Bellevue School of Medicine, and was graduated with honors in 1936, one of the first women to do so.

That was the year I was born, only a few miles away from Bellevue. When I allow myself such self-indulgent fantasies, I ponder whether God really did plant me on earth so that, almost half a century later and a continent away, I could meet the woman who cured cancer and help bring her convoluted and controversial story to the world at large.

4

Why Now? Why Then?

After so many years of battling the medical establishment, what made Dr. Virginia decide to write a book addressed to the American public? Exactly that: so many years of battling the establishment. In a word: frustration.

I got the impression more than once—indeed, on dozens of occasions—that after twenty-five years of trying to get independent corroboration that she was at least on the right track, Dr. Virginia had given up completely any thought of being acknowledged by the mainstream scientific community. Even after she discovered that the cancer microbe was Seitz filterable (thereby relating it in size to a virus) and began publishing scientific papers in respected journals, her theory was met with a deafening silence by her medical peers. Even after her microbe passed every test of Koch's postulates (the accepted foolproof scientific test that proves the cause of a disease; more on this and the Seitz filter later), medical authorities refused to examine her experiments. Even when, under a Fleet Foundation grant at the Biomed Laboratory of San Diego, she showed that her microbe not only caused cancerous degeneration of cells but also was sensitive to certain antibiotics, she was rebuked.

Why Not Then?

Dr. Virginia's papers and dissertations were published in respected journals that included the *American Journal of the Medical Sciences,* the *American Review of Respiratory Diseases,* the *Annals of the New York Academy of Sciences,* the *International Journal of Dermatology,* the *Journal of the American Medical Women's Association,* and the *Journal of the Medical Society of New Jersey,* among others. One of her papers was even presented at the historic meeting of the New York Academy of Sciences when, by invitation, she and her team classified her microorganism in the proper bacteriological fashion. All these were met with enthusiastic applause and commendation by assembled scientists and medical peers—but not officially by the medical establishment. (I once asked Dr. Virginia point blank why her papers and theories were not published in the highest echelon of medical and scientific journals such as the *Journal of the American Medical Association,* the *New England Medical Journal, Science, Lancet,* and a few others. Her reply, typical in its bluntness and implied obstinacy: "They want me to do double-blind studies. They forget that I've taken the same Hippocratic oath they have. Such a study would mean I'd have to withhold from half of my patients a treatment that I know to be effective, which is illegal, unethical, and immoral.")

So, after more than two decades of such scorn, Dr. Virginia decided to take her argument to the American public. Unfortunately, this meant translating her work into plain English, which Dr. Virginia wouldn't—or couldn't, really, by her very nature—let me do. In retrospect, I discovered that this left me between a rock and a hard spot: the "plain English" parts of *The Conquest of Cancer* were criticized by the medical community as being "not scientifically presented." And the technical parts of the narrative were unintelligible to the reading public.

But I digress.

Billions of dollars, maybe trillions, have been spent in the last half-century to determine the cause and cure for cancer. Despite this enormous funding, more than the collective cost of all the wars we've fought, cancer today is still on the increase. A mysterious "virus" is being sought in sophisticated research laboratories across the land, yet still hasn't been found. We've made remarkable strides in treating and curing *some* cancers, true. But overall, cancer is still considered a killer disease and its incidence is still on the rise.

Why is this so? Every quack with an apricot pit or a ray gun or a crystal pyramid or a magic stone from outer space gets a critical examination at some level of technical depth and ultimately a condemnation from medical authorities and government agencies. But not Dr. Virginia, with her sound scientific data; she was simply ignored. So the question the public should be asking is this: With all the money being spent over all the years by all the agencies and independent laboratories, why not investigate the *possibility* of a cure that has been postulated with some level of authority for half a century? Why not either prove her wrong or replicate her experiments? As we're seeing, there are "discoveries" being made today and described in scientific journals like broccoli sprouts (already mentioned in Chapter 2) that Dr. Virginia described sixty and seventy years ago. There are accepted treatments today like bacillus Calmette-Guerin (BCG) vaccine for bladder cancer that Dr. Virginia urged thirty-five years ago.

Why Now?

These are strong statements. Thirty-two years ago, Dr. Virginia decided to publish her findings for the American people to read about. She told me often (perhaps in tacit acknowledgment of having stubbornly burned many bridges behind her) that she was confident that after her death her theories would be validated. She steadfastly claimed that autogenous vaccines were powerful weapons against cancer, but that if no one accepted hers at the time, then a similar one would be formulated after her death (again, indirectly admitting that when she was "out of the way," maybe the medical community would get on with investigating her work).

That was in 1984. Fourteen years later, in 1998, yet another new study appeared. This one was conducted at the Massachusetts Institute of Technology's Whitehead Institute for Biomedical Research, and also published in the *Proceedings of the National Academy of Sciences*. It announced that by fusing a molecule from a patient's own tumor with a so-called heat shock protein, a vaccine (could it be called an autogenous vaccine?) can be made to mount a strong defense against the *infection* of cancer. (The importance of the word "infection" in the report cannot be overemphasized. When Dr. Virginia used the word in connection with cancer, she was figuratively laughed off the stage.)

Around 1910, Peyton Rous, M.D., demonstrated that 90 percent of chickens for sale in New York City were cancerous. He defined the poultry infection as caused by an unknown microbial agent that passed through a special filter designed to hold back bacteria, but not viruses (the Seitz filter). The filterability of this "cancer agent" led to the erroneous belief that cancer was caused by a virus, a belief held to this day almost a century later, but which Dr. Virginia always claimed that her own research proved was not true.

She formally classified her microbe as *Progenitor cryptocides* (more on this nomenclature later). She claimed to have isolated and cultured this bacterium, and made vaccines from it that were purported to have boosted the immunity of pre-cancer patients and put those with the disease into permanent remission. She claimed the disease was transmissible from animals to man, and that it may be present in our bodies from birth but suppressed by our immune systems. In her book, *The Conquest of Cancer,* she predicted that the science of immunotherapy would become the single most powerful anticancer program for all kinds of cancers. She said, "I predict that in ten years immunotherapy will be the prevailing treatment of cancer patients."

It appears she was short of the mark. It also appears she was short of the mark only by a few years.

5

Dr. Owen Wheeler's Story

Oone day during the preparation of Dr. Virginia's book, I sat down with Dr. Owen Webster Wheeler, Dr. Virginia's husband at the time I knew her (her fourth, including the seldom mentioned alcoholic Pulitzer journalist). A kind, gentle, God-fearing man highly respected in his community, he had offered me his own story as an example of the need for investigating new ideas before committing to a specific treatment for cancer.

Dr. Owen, as I came to call him, was a medical doctor who practiced in San Diego for thirty years, and was one of the founders of Doctors Hospital in that city. He told me that a few years before he met Dr. Virginia, he was shaving one morning when his wife noticed a lump on the side and toward the rear of his neck, just above the clavicle. He hadn't noticed it before and when he examined it himself, he became frightened. His medical training told him what it was, but he was quite frank in telling me that, at the time, he didn't want to admit it to himself. He commented to his wife that it was "peculiar," and promised her he'd have it looked at.

That very afternoon he consulted with a surgeon friend, to whom he had referred hundreds of patients from his family practice, and with whom he had assisted in hundreds of operations. The surgeon had a biopsy performed and a few days later handed Dr. Owen the grim report. There was no question that it was cancer. Worse, it was inoperable because it was attached to the carotid artery (which supplies blood to the brain) and wrapped around several important nerves and blood vessels.

Dr. Owen was shattered. He told me that his first reaction was to sit down in front of his friend and say absolutely nothing for a long time. Physicians, he said, when they start their medical practice and throughout their professional careers, take vaccinations and inoculations because they are exposed to disease all the time; usually, they stay well. Dr. Owen never thought he would get cancer, although he'd been around it so often. "What should I do? What should I do?" was all he could say. He was afraid.

His surgeon friend advised him that the standard radiation and chemotherapy techniques were his only hope since no one would operate. Without them, he said, Dr. Owen had no chance to survive for more than a year.

He recalled sitting down one evening and wondering whether he would be alive in a year, and whether, if he were, he'd only be a skeleton in some hospital bed. His wife and he cried. And they prayed.

Rejecting Useless "Cures"

A physician sees cancer all the time. They read about it, they see other doctors' patients, they discover it in their own patients, and they hear about it in the medical meetings they're always attending. And they almost always advise the orthodox treatments. They have to, of course. A physician could lose his license if he ordered an "unproved" cancer treatment other than surgery, radiation, or chemotherapy.

Dr. Owen finally called an old friend, a local oncologist to whom he'd referred many patients. The oncologist agreed with the surgeon: that the tumor, which was the size of a small lemon, was completely inoperable because it was surrounding so many nerves and blood vessels and was touching the top of one lung. Dr. Owen knew if this person couldn't "get it all," as they say, no one could, because he was one of the best.

Dr. Owen said he did a strange thing then. At least, he said, it seemed strange at the time of the telling. He had been referring cancer patients not only to this oncologist but also to several others for many years, and it suddenly occurred to him that he hadn't ever seen many of those patients again. He called the various specialists, and discovered that most of his patients had died. He thought of his father, who had died of cancer a number of years earlier. Nothing the doctors had done had been able to save his life. And the tragedy was that at the autopsy it was determined that there was no cancer left in him. He was rid of the cancer and had been killed by generalized infection due to immune suppression.

Dr. Owen decided that he didn't want to be treated with radiation or chemotherapy. It struck him as curious that for years he'd been referring patients for radiation and chemotherapy procedures, and now he was reluctant to undergo them himself. He had been recommending treatments that seldom cured! His vocal question to me was sincere: "Why do oncologists keep administering the same treatments over and over again when they rarely work?

Dr. Owen said he began to feel guilty. Why did he, a physician/ healer, recommend that his patients subject themselves to useless "cures"?

Investigating the Alternatives

He decided to investigate what was being done in alternative cancer therapy. He was looking for people who were doing something other than what he'd been advising for the past ten or fifteen years. He was only sixty-two at the time and wanted to live a few more years.

A friend finally said, "Why don't you look in your own backyard, Owen? There's the Livingston Clinic here in San Diego and they're doing something with cancer patients." He hadn't heard anything about the clinic. He called and made an appointment, and when he got there Dr. Virginia took his history. She commented on the fact that he was a physician who was willing to look at alternative therapies and pointed out that, at the time, there had only been a few other physicians to visit the clinic before him.

Dr. Virginia showed him around the laboratory, explained her work with the dark-field microscope, and gave him some of her published papers to read. He read about her pioneering work in microbiology and bacteriology, as well as her discoveries of the cancer-causing *Progenitor cryptocides* microbe and the hormone that it secreted. He finally saw the microbe in his own blood sample under the dark-field microscope. It was more exciting to him than anything an astronaut circling the moon could have imagined. He felt he was becoming a part of medical history.

As a physician, he had to admit that Dr. Virginia's approach was completely new to him. Nothing in the literature and the standard cancer information that was being published indicated that anyone was immunizing against cancer. Dr. Virginia explained in detail how the first vaccine—the bacillus Calmette-Guerin (BCG) that was developed for tuberculosis and that she claimed was a first cousin to her own *P. cryptocides* bacillus)—was also effective against cancer when used with her other modalities and how it was possible that by treating his own total immune system that cancer was a do-it-yourself-treatment disease that his own body could fight—but only if his immune system could be strengthened. She also explained that she made an autogenous vaccine from the actual microbe cultured from his own body fluids. He suddenly realized that he was placing his life in the hands of a woman who claimed to have discovered that cancer was caused by a bacterium, not a virus as he had been taught in medical school. He realized a lot of what she was telling him went totally against his professional training. He, and almost every other doctor in the land, had always stated that it was impossible to have such a bug in one's blood and still live.

After looking at the whole treatment process with an open mind, Dr. Owen decided that it made good scientific sense, and he consented to undergo the program. Within five months his tumor was completely gone. At the time of our meeting, in 1983, there had never been any recurrence, and it had now been more than ten years. He swore he hadn't been sick a day since.

(See "Taking Charge," below, for a cancer survivor's tips on how like Dr. Owen to ferret out everything about the cancer and the best possible treatment for it.)

"Keeping such a binder may be obvious to some people," Steve

TAKING CHARGE: A BREAST CANCER DIARY

There are right things and wrong things to do when someone is diagnosed with cancer. Some people panic. Some give up immediately and do nothing. Some do whatever a doctor—*one* doctor—tells them. Some seek legitimate alternative paths to recovery, and some go for goofy and unproved regimens only offered in foreign countries. And some, like Steven and Carrie Rosenberg, dedicate themselves to finding out everything they possibly can about the cancer and discovering the best possible treatment for it.

When Steve and Carrie found out she had breast cancer, Steve set out to find out every option for treating it, every doctor who specialized in it, and all of the latest technologies for analyzing it. During the entire process, he kept a copious notebook, cross-indexed, and neatly tabulated, which eventually became the most complete "How-to-Deal-with-It Manual" I've ever seen.

"You have to become your own general contractor," Steve advises. "You have to select the best people for the job, and to do that you have to interview everyone who qualifies and remember everything that's been said."

Steve also advises what I've heard from many other victims of not only cancer, but also of several other life-threatening conditions: the patient has to have an advocate. Ideally, this should be a person somewhat knowledgeable about things medical—a nurse, say—but usually someone close to the patient who shares a deep concern for what's happening and for the patient's ultimate well-being. A spouse, a close friend, a close relative—someone who has the time and devotion to attend every meeting and appointment the patient has, and listen in on every conversation—even phone calls—the patient makes, all the while taking diligent notes and asking pertinent questions.

"Many patients facing cancer are too emotionally traumatized to remember important facts or instructions, or even to ask the right questions," Steve says. "The patient advocate must become part of the patient's brain."

Steve, a lawyer, assembled two large 3-ring binders, one to record the day-to-day history of research, investigative results, appointments, and so on; and the other to store articles and printed information concerning, in this case, breast cancer. The binder was constantly within arm's reach.

The binder is divided into eight sections:

1. **To do:** A running tally of appointments and lists of things to attend to soon, a list of books to read, CDs to watch, tapes to acquire and listen to, etc. It also listed treatment options to investigate, which is one of the first priorities a cancer patient should set.

2. **Phone numbers:** A complete list of available physicians, clinics, specialists, and others, even acupuncturists, and their phone numbers. It also had a page with a list of every friend's and relative's phone number, and another page with a meticulously organized telephone tree.

3. **Notes and correspondence:** A list of appointments, with entries such as "August 2, 1999: Bone Density Test" or "April 26, 2000: Mammogram." Another page kept a complete chronology of Carrie's disease, from the discovery of the lump to her last MRI. This section also had a compendium, both typed and in long hand, of the notes from every doctor's visit and treatment Carrie had. An example: "(Dr.'s name and phone number). Diagnosis: lobular carcinoma. The location is

insignificant in terms of how it acts. It is at least 5 cm. Exact size is difficult to determine with a lobular carcinoma. It's hard to tell where it starts and stops. Therefore not sure they got it all when they did the lumpectomy." The report also discussed growth rate and treatment regimen—all the result of Steve's attentive note taking during the visit.

4. **Reports:** Copies of every lab report, patient analysis, screening, radiology, pathology and MRI report. It even had copies of sketches various specialists had drawn to illustrate Carrie's condition.

5. **Doctors:** Information about every doctor available for Carrie's condition, including treatment centers throughout California and nearby states.

6. **Resources and support groups:** Notes on diet, medications, alternative therapies, including several daily diaries of Carrie's post-treatment reactions and side effects of radiation, chemotherapy, etc.

7. **Insurance:** Cancer treatment is expensive, and patients should know all their payment and reimbursement options.

8. **Diet and medications:** Everything Steve could learn about diets for cancer patients, and a regimen for changing the family diet accordingly, such as adding more cruciferous vegetables and reducing alcohol intake. It also contained a running chart of Carrie's blood pressure and a continuing list of her medications and dosages.

says, "but its main purpose is to keep a day-to-day record of a patient's disease-related activities, and to keep the advocate organized."

Through the ordeal Carrie had two lumpectomies, a Tamoxifen course, a mastectomy, Chinese medicine regimens, post-op chemo courses, active support group attendance and a cheerful, positive outlook.

Today Carrie has been happily back at work and cancer free for ten years.

From Patient to Work Partner and Husband

Shortly after Dr. Owen's first meeting with Dr. Virginia in 1975, her husband, Dr. A. M. Livingston, died. Dr. Owen's wife had died recently of heart disease. Six months after Dr. Virginia's husband died, she called Dr. Owen to ask if he could come and help her run the clinic. The burden of running it single-handedly was too much, and she would have had to close it had she been unable to find another physician suitable to help out. He was then the only doctor who understood what she was doing and who had seen her results firsthand.

He told Dr. Virginia not to close the clinic, that he would help. Any program that could cure him the way it did was bound to help other patients. He started working at the clinic part-time and devoting less and less time to running his own practice. He eventually became so busy at the clinic that he finally resigned from his partnership to work full-time at the clinic. Dr. Virginia and he kept the clinic open, working side by side, continually treating cancer patients and watching them get well. He told me he was also greatly impressed with Dr. Virginia's unexcelled compassion and concern for her patients.

A year later they were married.

6

An Attempt
to Be Objective

Whenever Dr. Virginia gave a lecture to a professional group—
at least the ones at which I was present—she was invariably
asked for statistics to back up her claims of success. Also invariably,
her reply was that she had been too experimentally involved with
her ongoing program to offer an overall statistical study of her
patients for public release. But also, she felt that a double-blind
response (which requires withholding treatment from half of her
patients), as previously mentioned, would be a violation of her Hippocratic oath.

She also tried to explain to her audiences the complex problem
of quantifying many different conditions for comparison with each
other. That is, how does one compare a rectal tumor that has metastasized to the liver in a thirty-year-old male with a single small lump
in the breast of a sixty-year-old female requiring a simple lumpectomy? Suppose the latter patient adopts Dr. Virginia's program and
becomes completely clear with no recurrence of the tumor, while
the other patient adopts the program, has the tumor removed, dis-
covers the lesion has disappeared, but then drops the program and
has a recurrence? How do you compare the two cases? Two remissions? One remission and one failure? And what about the biochemical differences in each person's makeup? What about DNA?
Genetics? Diet? Ancestral history?

In other words, Dr. Virginia always insisted that a statistical survey of her patients would be inconclusive. However, she never failed to cap off her explanation with a passionate invitation to *anyone* or *any agency* to visit her clinic and do an independent survey and analysis.

Our Own Statistical Study

Considering all this, once we agreed to do her book I insisted on *some* kind of attempt at objectivity. Knowing full well the skeptical reception the book would get in mainstream medical circles, and understanding that it was to be, after all, a book for the lay reader, I suggested that a third party select 100 random charts from her files. Such a random selection, I reasoned, would preclude any suspicion of our having presented only the most positive of her cases for analysis.

Dr. Virginia agreed. She picked one of her assistants to do the random selection, but I objected immediately. Not even someone she knew, I insisted. It must be a third party with whom neither of us was acquainted, someone totally unknown to either Dr. Virginia or her staff.

Again she agreed. At dinner that evening, we defined specific ground rules that I, albeit an amateur statistician, thought would provide our random case history review with optimally credible methodology. They were:

1. All patients in the study were to have had their diagnoses made by a qualified pathologist who had examined the tissue under a microscope, before coming to the clinic.

2. If a patient selected was *not* a cancer patient—that is, had come to the clinic for hepatitis or allergies, or some affliction not related to cancer—we would exclude the chart.

3. If a patient had come to the clinic against the wishes of his or her physician, and then after leaving the clinic was dissuaded by the

physician from continuing the program and discontinued the vaccines in favor of resuming chemotherapy and radiation, then their case was excluded.

4. All patients were excluded who "went home to die," that is, who were too weak or debilitated to carry out the program, or who simply gave up their will to live.

5. All patients who were too new to the program to have shown any results at all (six months or less) were also excluded.

The next day we approached the clinic's bottled-water delivery-man and he volunteered to help. We watched as he carefully paced back and forth before the clinic's multi-tiered files of patient charts, plucking them out at random until we had 100. According to the regimen I had laid out, we then took the charts home, went over each according to our criteria, and were left with 62 charts.

Next, I insisted that Dr. Virginia personally contact every patient represented by our sample, or their physician, to ascertain their current status.

It took three days to make all 62 connections, either with the patient, his or her physician, or a knowledgeable relative. Here are the totals of the study:

Seventeen of the 62 cases we selected had been officially diagnosed as "terminal" when they appeared at the clinic's door. Four cases had died or were presumed dead. The types of cancer broke down as follows:

- Breast (5)
- Breast and lung(s) (4)
- Breast and nodes (8)
- Breast and rib(s) (3)
- Breast and uterus (1)
- Colon (3)
- Colon and liver (3)
- Esophagus (1)
- Hodgkin's lymphoma (6)
- Kidney (1)

- Kidney and liver (1)
- Larynx (1)
- Lung and liver (2)
- Lung and neck, oat-cell (1)
- Lung and nodes (2)
- Melanomas (6)
- Ovaries and colon (1)
- Ovaries and nodes (1)
- Ovaries and uterus (1)
- Pancreatic and liver (1)
- Pelvic (1)
- Prostate (3)
- Skin, basal cell (2)
- Uterus (1)
- Uterus and liver (2)
- Uterus and rectum (1)

My examination of the 62 cases showed that the clinic's success rate was 82 percent. Dr. Virginia insisted that, considering the patients she called "inconclusive" but for whom she was able to offer *some* degree of recovery or comfort, it was more like 90 percent.

Dr. Virginia went on to compare our figures with the "official" American Cancer Society figure of patients who, as of 1983, were helped by radiation and chemotherapy. (It should also be noted that the two physicians in our random survey elected not to be treated by either radiation or chemotherapy; I found this to be true of most physician-patients who visited the clinic.)

Dr. Virginia also insisted at the time that the patients who had died or were presumed dead would not have done so if they had not appeared at the clinic with enormously debilitated immune systems as a result of previous radiation and/or chemotherapy.

Findings from Sixty-Two Case Histories

When her book was published, this list of case histories was met with a barrage of criticism. Some critics either didn't read my explanation of how we selected the charts, or else they wanted to believe Dr. Virginia "salted" the results and so they didn't believe us. Other skeptics thought we simply made up the list. Still others, especially physicians, thought we didn't describe the cases in enough depth, or with enough medical accuracy. I regret this, because they were probably right. I didn't have the control I wanted in presenting the cases on paper, and I suppose I was also naive enough at the time not to have asked the in-depth questions that would have made the case histories more acceptable to the medical professionals. In any event, I accept the criticism, even today, and offer no apology or excuse other than when I tried to make the case histories more technical and medically complete, they were unintelligible to the reading public, and when I tried to present them in plain English, they were too simplistic (and Dr. Virginia, who, as I said, only spoke "Bacteriology," wouldn't accept them). So, they were eventually published as a peculiar form of "pidgin-medicine."

Nevertheless, whatever the critics chose to believe then—and choose to believe today—I will swear under oath that the case histories were absolutely selected at random by a disinterested third party, and when we telephoned the patients and their families I made it a point to speak to each and every one of them myself to verify their identity.

Moreover, what is not stated in each case history, but was a prerequisite as stated above, is that each patient's condition was diagnosed by a pathologist who had examined the tissue under a microscope, and that each diagnosis was duly recorded in the patient's chart.

Here were the results as published in her book back in 1984 (slightly annotated for clarity). In some cases "at the time of this writing" means the fall of 1983. "We" refers not to Dr. Virginia and me, but to her and her staff at the Livingston-Wheeler Clinic.

TERMS OF CANCER

Adenoma. Benign glandular tumor.

Adenocarcinoma. A type of cancer that forms in the mucous-secreting glands throughout the body.

Apoptosis. Programmed cell death.

Basal cell cancer. The most common type of skin cancer originating from pigment cells in the outer layer of the skin.

Carcinogenesis. The process by which normal cells are transformed into cancer cells.

Carcinoma. A malignant tumor that begins in the epithelial tissues (the cells that line the entire surface of the body); approximately 80 percent of all cancers are carcinomas.

Differentiation. How normal or abnormal the cancer cells look under a microscope; tumor cells that are well differentiated and are similar in appearance to normal cells tend to be less aggressive than cells that are poorly differentiated.

Grade. The degree of a cancer's severity; the lower the grade, the less advanced the cancer and the greater the chance for cure.

Human choriogonadotropin (HCG). A hormone found in abundance in all human tumors.

Hyperplasia. Excessive growth of cells.

Infiltrating cancer. Invasive. Cancer that can grow beyond its site of origin into neighboring tissue.

Intraductal. Within the duct. Intraductal can describe a benign or malignant process.

Lesion. An area of abnormal tissue.

Level. A term used to describe the depth of a tumor rather than its length.

Lymphoma. A cancer involving the lymphatic system.

Melanoma. A malignant tumor originating from pigment cells in the deep layers of the skin.

Metastasis. The spread of cancer to a site or sites away from the original tumor.

Neoplasm. An abnormal growth.

Nodes. Glands located along the lymphatic system that help defend against foreign invaders such as bacteria.

Node-positive. An indication that cancer cells have been found in the lymph nodes.

Sarcoma. A malignant tumor that grows from connective tissue such as cartilage, fat, muscle, or bone.

Staging. A way to categorize or classify patients according to how extensive the disease is at the time of diagnosis. Stage I indicates the earliest cancers. Stages II, III, and IV indicate progressively more extensive disease. Letters may be used along with the numerals (Stage IIB, for example) to subclassify cancers based on specific tumor characteristics. *See* Grade.

Tumor. Abnormal mass of tissue.

1. **A fifty-three-year old female** came to the clinic in January 1978 with cancer of the right breast and metastasis to the spine and pelvis. A mastectomy had been done ten years earlier on the left breast, and a pin had been placed in her leg after it had broken from metastasis. She had undergone several courses of chemotherapy but had decided to stop when lesions continued to grow. We placed her on our standard program of immunotherapy. In January 1983, a bone scan showed she was completely clear. Our telephone follow-up at the time revealed she had returned to work and felt well.

2. **A fifty-six-year-old female** came to the clinic in January 1981 with recurrent intraductal cancer of the right breast. She had had a left mastectomy in 1980, with six positive nodes and a thyroid nodule removed. Follow-up chemotherapy had not prevented a recurrence of another malignant lymph node, and the patient elected to come to the clinic rather than have a second surgery. We placed her on the standard program of immunotherapy. Echograms at the end of 1982 showed she was clear of cancer. A bone scan was also negative in 1982, and a visit to the clinic shortly before I (EGA) arrived showed that she was still clear.

3. **A forty-year-old male** came to the clinic in November 1981, after leaving the Mayo Clinic. His pathology report indicated nodular sclerosing Hodgkin's disease (a form of glandular cancer). He received the standard program of immunotherapy and then had the nodules removed by surgery while staying on his immune program. After immunotherapy he had a further precautionary course of radiation, a laparotomy, and a splenectomy, at which time he was told he was free of disease. A radiology report at the time indicated that he was clear of cancer and when we called he said he was leading a normal life.

4. **A fifty-nine-year-old female** came to the clinic in September

1976 with a pathology report of a right radical mastectomy indicating intraductal cancer. She had no previous radiation or chemotherapy. She received our usual program in addition to having several small, left supraclavicular (above the collarbone) nodes excised. At the time we called her, she remained cancer free and was on the clinic's preventive program (a modified version of Dr. Virginia's standard program of immunotherapy).

5. **A fifty-nine-year-old female** came to the clinic in October 1973 with a pathology report of basal cell carcinoma of the lip and low-grade cancer of the thyroglossal duct. She had a pelvic complaint. Since cancer is multi-local, she had dilatation and curettage (D&C) of the uterus, which detected severe hyperplasia of the lining of the uterus. She was put on the usual program with additional preventive vaccines. A telephone check at the time indicated she was still clear of cancer and feeling well after local follow-up.

6. **A fifty-two-year-old female** came to the clinic in March 1981 with a history of cancer of the left breast and metastatic cancer of the lung. She had had a radical mastectomy and radiation for recurrent disease, confirmed by pathology as infiltrating ductal adenocarcinoma. Her diagnosis was labeled "advanced terminal." At the time she responded well to immunotherapy. A chest examination in January 1983 indicated she was stabilized with no advancing lesions and when we called her she had returned to work.

7. **A fifty-three-year-old female** came to the clinic in October 1980 with eight out of ten positive nodes after a mastectomy in 1979. Post-operatively, she had received radiation for twenty-three days and chemotherapy courses for one year. When her nodes returned she came to the clinic and was put on the standard program of immunotherapy. Her nodes diminished. However, she suddenly dropped out of the program and left the clinic. Five

months later she returned to the clinic with an abdominal tumor. Diagnosis revealed a 3-centimeter (cm) mass (1.2 inches [in]) of bilateral metastatic cancer of both ovaries. We started her on the standard program again and referred her for surgical removal of her ovaries. Echograms indicated she was clear of cancer following our treatment and surgery. A telephone check at the time indicated she had had no recurrence and she reported she was feeling well.

8. **A sixty-four-year-old female** came to the clinic in August 1974 with Level III malignant melanoma of the left ankle and groin resection. She responded well to immunotherapy. Tests in 1982 indicated she remained cleared of cancer. She returned for regular checkups and when I contacted her during our follow-ups, she reported that she was still clear.

9. **A sixty-five-year-old male** came to the clinic in May 1981 with cancer of the prostate with multiple metastases to the bone (revealed by scan in 1980). On the standard program his prostate mass had gone down by July 1981, and his bone lesions greatly diminished by August 1982. A check with his physician at the time we wrote the book indicated he was doing well, continuing his vaccines and diet program.

10. **A thirty-three-year-old female** came to the clinic in January 1979 with a diagnosis of Hodgkin's disease. She had had earlier surgical removal of a mass in her right lung, but when she came to the clinic periaortic nodules (around the aorta) were present. She responded well to the standard program of immunotherapy and at the time her chart was pulled she had remained clear for the past four years. At the time of our follow-up telephone call, we found she'd undergone considerable emotional trauma recently when she'd discovered a recurrence in her chest. Dr. Virginia scheduled her for a course of modified chemotherapy while re-instituting an immunotherapy program.

I did not follow up on her after the book was published.

11. **A fifty-one-year-old male** came to the clinic in February 1977 with Level II malignant melanoma of the nodular type in his back, as well as aortic nodes. He had had multiple surgeries to remove the nodes. Even after continued recurrences, he responded well to immunotherapy. Radiology reports in February 1983 confirmed that there was no evidence of cancer in his body.

12. **A sixty-eight-year-old female** who came to the clinic from New York in September 1980 with tumors of the uterus, a 7 cm (2.7 in) tumor of the vagina, and lesions of the liver. She weighed 80 pounds and was a total invalid. After immunization, Dr. Virginia referred her to a local hospital in San Diego for small doses of chemotherapy and radiation. Ultrasound and scans in February 1981 indicated the tumor and lesions were diminishing. She returned to New York. When we called her physician he indicated that, while not completely clear, she was recovering well, weighed 120 pounds, and had resumed her career.

13. **A sixty-seven-year-old female** came to the clinic in June 1976 with a pathology report of two positive masses in her breasts. She had refused a mastectomy, but after diagnosis at the clinic we recommended surgical removal of the masses, followed by the standard program of immunotherapy. When she returned to the clinic in February 1983 for tests, she was still clear.

14. **A sixty-three-year-old female** came to the clinic in June 1972 for preventive care following radiation and a right radical mastectomy with two positive nodes. In 1975 she developed hypercalcemia (an excess of calcium in the blood). A parathyroid adenoma was found and surgically removed. She had had no recurrence and at the time we contacted her she remained well.

15. **A thirty-eight-year-old female** came to the clinic in February

1974 with widespread cancer of the abdomen following surgery in January 1973 for adenocarcinoma and bilateral involvement of the ovaries with attachment to the uterus. Radiation followed surgery, but the cancer had spread to her scarred underlying tissue. At the clinic she followed the immunotherapy program. In 1978 ultrasound showed no metastases, no fluid, and that her liver was clear; a chest x-ray in 1981 was normal. A pelvic examination and echograms during a recent follow-up visit to the clinic showed she was still clear of cancer. A phone call verified this.

16. **A fifty-five-year-old female** came to the clinic in June 1976 with a diagnosis of terminal lymphoma, Hodgkin's disease. Pleural effusion and a periaortic node, measuring 6 by 5 cm (2.3 by 1.9 in), were present, as well as liver metastasis. She underwent immunotherapy and stabilized in 1978. Echograms in 1980 indicated that she was free of cancer, and her nodes normal. In 1982 ultrasound indicated her liver was normal with no masses. A recent office visit at the time we wrote the book revealed she was still clear of cancer but had developed cardiac angina and heart disease. A phone call verified this.

17. **A seventy-six-year-old female** came to the clinic in March 1976 after a radical mastectomy for poorly differentiated carcinoma of the breast, followed by four out of twelve nodes tested positive for cancer. She underwent the standard program of immunotherapy, and by the end of 1976 a complete checkup indicated that she was clear. A telephone report at the time indicated she is was healthy and doing well. She received no radiation or chemotherapy.

18. **A sixty-six-year-old male** came to the clinic in June 1978 with inoperable cancer of the right kidney with metastasis to the liver and a massive retro-peritoneal lesion from the liver to the pelvis. He had received some radiation but stopped it and came to the

clinic. He received the immunotherapy program and by 1979 he was feeling much better. In 1980 his tumor had diminished from 8 to 4 cm (3 to 1.5 in). By 1981 his cancer had stabilized. A telephone check at the time indicated he was still on his program and doing well.

19. **A forty-one-year-old male** came to the clinic in August 1973 with a diagnosis of Level IV melanoma of the right thigh with metastatic nodes in the groin removed by surgery. He responded well to the standard program of immunotherapy. A biopsy in January of 1983 at the University of California, Los Angeles, indicated he was still totally free of cancer. When we called him from Dr. Virginia's home, he was still clean.

20. **A fifty-year-old female** who came to the clinic in June of 1977 with infiltrative lobular carcinoma of the right breast and two positive axillary (armpit) nodes. She had refused both surgery and chemotherapy. We put her on the standard program of immunotherapy. Echograms in 1979 showed that she was totally clear. However, while traveling for two years she went off the program and relapsed. She returned to the clinic in 1981 with cancer spread to the chest wall and pathological confirmation of positive neck nodes. She resumed the immunotherapy program, and echograms conducted just before the time we wrote the book showed that she was clear once again.

21. **A twenty-one-year-old male** who came to the clinic in January 1976 with Hodgkin's disease, positive nodes in the neck, and metastasis to the bone. He had undergone three courses of chemotherapy during a four-month period, but stopped treatments prior to arriving at the clinic. He had also had his spleen removed. We treated him with the standard program of immunotherapy. An ultrasound in 1981 showed him clear of metastases. The last time he was seen for examination at the clinic, in September 1982, all scans were negative.

22. **A seventy-two-year-old female** came to the clinic in August 1974 with malignant melanoma on her back and positive nodes under the left arm. She underwent our standard program of immunotherapy. An ultrasound in 1981 showed her clean, and echograms and scans in May 1982 indicated she was still clean with no recurrence. A visit to the clinic just prior to the time of this writing showed her still clear.

23. **A seventy-one-year-old male** came to the clinic in November 1977 following removal of a tumor of the colon and a pathology report showing positive nodes with metastasis to the omentum (a fatty "apron" extending from the stomach along the abdominal wall and covering the intestines). He responded well to the standard program of immunotherapy. An ultrasound in 1980 showed no evidence of new lesions and no enlargements of old lesions. A phone call to his family physician at the time of this writing confirms he is clear and feeling well.

24. **A sixty-nine-year-old female** came to the clinic in December 1975 with a pathological diagnosis of poorly differentiated adenocarcinoma of the breast with metastasis to surrounding nodes following a modified mastectomy the previous year. She refused further surgery and underwent our standard program of immunotherapy. A bone scan was negative in 1981. Regular office checkups up to the time of this writing confirm she is still clear with no recurrence.

25. **A fifty-five-year-old female** came to the clinic in September 1979 with squamous cell carcinoma of the larynx confirmed by biopsy. We referred her for mild radiation and gave her simultaneous immunization with the standard program of immunotherapy. A laryngoscopic examination of her throat in April 1982 showed no malignancy.

26. **A sixty-one-year-old female** came to the clinic in April 1980 with a pathology report of Grade III intraductal cell carcinoma

NEWS UPDATE:
TOMATOES AT HARVARD

Dr. Virginia was ridiculed for including a strict cruciferous vegetarian diet and vitamin regimen in her multimodal immunotherapy treatment of cancer patients, but the beat goes on. In 2002, after a nine-year study of 48,000 men, Edward Giovannucci, M.D., of Harvard Medical School stated in the *Journal of the National Cancer Institute* that eating tomatoes "is an effective way to reduce the risk of prostate cancer." The antioxidant agent lycopene, a red carotenoid pigment, also present in strawberries, watermelon, and papaya, is the effective ingredient.

According to Dr. Giovannucci's study, consuming tomato sauce, marinara sauce, tomato paste, and tomato juice can protect against prostate cancer by preventing free radicals. His research said tomato servings were associated with a 35 percent reduced risk of prostate cancer. And according to William Nelson, M.D., of the Brady Urological Institute at Johns Hopkins University, the lycopenes actually enter the prostate gland. "You can't say that about everything you swallow," he is quoted as saying in *Prostate Cancer Update*.

In 2012, research published in the *British Journal of Nutrition* reported that Mridula Chopra, Ph.D., and her colleagues at the University of Portsmouth, United Kingdom, tested the effect of lycopene on the simple mechanism through which cancer cells hijack a body's healthy blood supply to grow and spread. They found that lycopene intercepts a cancer's ability to make the connections it needs to attach to a healthy blood supply. The researchers said, "This simple chemical reaction was shown to occur at lycopene concentrations that can easily be achieved by eating processed tomatoes."

Makes you wonder about prostate cancer in Italians, doesn't it? Well, one Japanese study published in the *Japanese Journal of Clinical Oncology* (2010) states, "the age-standardized rates of prostate cancer among males from the United States, United Kingdom, and France were similar, while those among Italian men tended to be lower." In 1995, an

Australian study of Aussies and Italian immigrants reported in *Cancer Causes & Control* had found the mortality rate from prostate cancer markedly lower in the Italian immigrants. In a breakdown of the estimated 12.7 million new cases, age-standardized incidence rates and the most commonly diagnosed cancers by the different regions of the world, the World Health Organization *Global Status Report* cited in 2008 that Spain and Italy had the lowest percentage of prostate cancers.

It should also be noted that the lycopene compound is described as a carotenoid pigment. Human beings possess four carotenoids: alpha-carotene, beta-carotene, gamma-carotene, and beta-cryptoxanthin—all of which can be converted to retinol, which is one of the many forms of . . . guess what? Vitamin A.

and metastasis to the right lobe of the liver. She had had a lumpectomy in March 1980 and refused further surgery, radiation, and chemotherapy. We treated her with the standard program of immunotherapy and as of October 1982 echograms showed she was clear of cancer. Telephone follow-up at the time of this writing confirmed she is still well.

27. **A twenty-five-year-old male** came to the clinic in June 1976 with Hodgkin's disease and 128 subcutaneous skin lesions of his neck and back, complicated by severe allergies. He responded well when treated with immunotherapy plus surgical removal of some of the nodes. Unfortunately, he refused to maintain his program of vaccines and diet but came back to the clinic whenever he discovered a new lesion, at which point the clinic reinstituted his program. At his last visit prior to the time of this writing, he had a small lesion in the supraclavicular left neck, now receding. His health is otherwise good.

28. **A forty-three-year-old male** came to the clinic in January 1981 for preventive therapy after surgery for the removal of a can-

cerous kidney. He responded well to our standard program of immunotherapy. He was seen in July 1982, and there was no further incidence of cancer.

29. **A sixty-seven-year-old male** came to the clinic in February 1982 with a huge 18 by 22 cm (7 by 8 in) chondrosarcoma of the right buttock. He had had radiation and chemotherapy, but the mass had continued to grow. At the clinic we referred him for surgical removal and treated him with immunotherapy. A recent check confirms that there has been no recurrence, and that he is completely normal.

30. **A twelve-year-old male** came to the clinic in April 1981 with advanced Hodgkin's disease after his mother had refused chemotherapy for him. He had developed a heart murmur and a lesion on his liver. We instituted an immunotherapy program but the court was threatening to take the child away from his mother because she had refused the chemotherapy. I informed the court that he was under our care; the mother was then allowed to keep him. In January 1982 an ultrasound indicated lymphoma in remission. A recent check confirmed that he is totally clear, back in school, gaining weight, and at the time of this writing has made the basketball team.

31. **A fifty-one-year-old female** came to the clinic in February 1981 with cancer of the ovaries and metastasis of an apple-sized tumor on the colon, which had been surgically removed. She also had a small node on the back of her neck removed. She had had 3,000 rads of radiation and two treatments of chemotherapy. She stopped the chemotherapy treatments because she was so sick. Her physician's report at the time she came to the clinic described her as "terminal." We treated her with immunotherapy, and in 1982 a pelvic and abdominal computerized axial tomography (CAT) scan was negative and an ultrasound was normal. At the time of this writing all scans were negative, and she was back to work.

32. **A sixty-seven-year-old female** came to the clinic in June 1977 with adenocarcinoma of the endometrium (the mucous membrane lining the uterus) with metastasis to the liver and having had a hysterectomy and radiation. A postoperative biopsy report revealed eight lesions approximately 4 by 4 cm (1.5 by 1.5 in) in the right lobe of the liver and positive nodes in the inguinal (groin) region. The patient refused further surgery and was treated with our program. As of October 1979, both nodes and liver lesions were proved cleared by scans. Telephone checkup at the time of this writing indicated she is still clear.

33. **A sixty-seven-year-old male** came to the clinic in May 1979 with cancer of the pancreas and metastasis to the liver. He had originally been admitted to the hospital with severe abdominal pain. Initial studies showed it to be pancreatitis, but an upper gastrointestinal series then revealed evidence of a mass lesion. A CAT scan showed a fairly extensive tumor of the pancreas involving the liver. The patient was told he had six weeks to live. He refused chemotherapy and came to the clinic. We treated him with immunotherapy and in May 1981 CAT, bone, and liver scans showed the tumor was in remission and the liver lesion decreased. A biopsy in February 1982 showed the liver normal.

34. **A forty-four-year-old female** came to the clinic in January 1981 with Paget's disease of the breast and bleeding from the nipple. (Paget's disease of the breast is a rare type of cancer of the nipple-areola area often associated with an underlying invasive carcinoma.) She had refused removal of the breast and underwent our program of immunotherapy. The surface of the nipple cleared but a biopsy revealed some malignant cells. She was still undecided whether to have a mastectomy, as urged by her oncologist in early 1983. A telephone check at the time of this writing revealed she had had the mastectomy, which showed her breast and axilla completely clear with only a few superficial neoplastic cells.

35. **A forty-three-year-old female** came to the clinic in January 1977 after discovering a nodule in her right breast. It was diagnosed as malignant and a mastectomy recommended. The patient preferred a lumpectomy, which she had. Afterward, we treated her with our program of immunotherapy, but she discontinued it. In January 1978 she had a recurrence and a mastectomy. A pathology report revealed an infiltrating ductal-type carcinoma with five out of twelve positive nodes in the axilla, estrogen positive, and an ovarian tumor. She had a modified hysterectomy and an oophorectomy (removal of the ovaries) in 1979 after resuming immunotherapy at the clinic. In February 1982 a mammogram showed no further metastases and no new nodes.

36. **A fifty-two-year-old female** came to the clinic in March 1980 following a hysterectomy for adenocarcinoma of the uterus with postoperative diagnosis of bilateral metastases to the pelvis and omentum. She could not take BCG vaccinations because of a positive skin test, but we treated her with autogenous vaccines and antibiotics, intravenous vitamin C, and diet therapy, standard in our immunotherapy program. She cleared by April 1981. In May of 1982 ultrasound showed there was no evidence of mass or lesions. Telephone follow-up right before writing the book verified continued good health.

37. **A seventy-three-year-old male** came to the clinic in October 1977 following removal of the upper lobe of the right lung for cancer, with a subsequent pathology report showing metastasis to the peribronchial lymph nodes and to the liver. He received our program of immunotherapy and in March 1979 x-rays, ultrasound, scans, and blood chemistry showed he was completely free of cancer. He continues to be clear at the time of this writing.

38. **A forty-eight-year-old female** came to the clinic in September 1978 with part of her liver and one-third of her colon removed. She was reported to have residual metastases. We treated her

with our program of immunotherapy, and in 1979 she stabilized. In December 1981 an ultrasound showed a normal liver and no evidence of cancer in the colon. A telephone conversation at the time of this writing indicated she is still clear.

39. **A thirty-seven-year-old female** came to the clinic in June 1981 with recurring tumors in the pelvic region. She had had pelvic masses, which were biopsied as lymphomas in 1976 with surgical removal followed by three and a half years of chemotherapy. When tumors continued to grow, she stopped the chemotherapy and we treated her with our program of immunotherapy. One year later, ultrasound showed the tumors had decreased. At the time of this writing, ultrasound showed a total absence of any masses and that she is free of cancer.

40. **A sixty-four-year-old female** came to the clinic in August 1981 with advanced cancer of the breast and twenty-eight positive nodes and metastasis to the bone and liver. An intensive immunotherapy program stabilized her, but the clinic suddenly lost contact with her. A telephone check with a close relative at the time of this writing indicated she had stopped her vaccines and diet in May 1982 and had died peacefully in her sleep of heart failure at the end of that year.

41. **A sixty-year-old male** came to the clinic in July 1975 having had a resection for cancer of the colon. He had metastasis to the liver and spine. This patient was a medical doctor who refused chemotherapy and radiation when he appeared at our clinic. We treated him with immunotherapy. A telephone check at the time of this writing confirmed that he is still completely recovered and active in his retirement. (Because he was a physician, I asked him if we could use his name for a more expanded case history in the book, but he refused permission—EGA.)

42. **A sixty-year-old female** came to the clinic in August 1979, referred to us as "terminal" by her doctor, who had given her

two to three weeks to live. She suffered from cancer of the esophagus and liver metastasis. She had had part of her stomach removed and nine months of chemotherapy. We treated her with immunotherapy, and at the time of this writing, three and a half years later, she is still alive, has gained five pounds, and is doing well. She reported that a recent CAT scan was negative, with no signs of cancer.

43. **A sixty-seven-year-old male** came to the clinic in October 1981 with metastatic cancer of the prostate, bones, bladder, and a large chest mass with rib destruction and right lung involvement. We treated him with immunotherapy, and at the time of this writing all scans are negative. His own physician also reports all cancer signs clear and scans negative.

44. **A seventy-year-old female** came to the clinic in November 1981, having had a mastectomy for infiltrating carcinoma of the left breast. We treated her preventively with the standard program of immunotherapy, and at the time of this writing she is still on the program and free of cancer.

45. **A seventy-one-year-old female** came to the clinic in July 1977 with a twenty-year history of recurring basal cell carcinoma on her face that had been periodically removed with cauterizations and surgeries. We put her on a prevention program. Except for two growths removed in October and December of 1981, she has had no recurrences. She continues with a modified immunotherapy program.

46. **A sixty-three-year-old female** came to the clinic in August 1981, diagnosed as "terminal" by her physician after having had colon surgery the previous March with a postoperative pathology report of widespread metastasis to the bones and an additional 4 cm (1.5 in) mass recurring on the colon. We treated her with immunotherapy, and at the time of this writing her scans

are still positive. She has had a recent colostomy and will have to have radiation. We are hopeful she will continue to survive.

47. **A forty-three-year-old female** came to the clinic in August 1979 with recurring nodules after having had modified mastectomies of the right breast in January and the left breast in July. She had come for preventive treatment and underwent our program. Tests at the end of August 1982 showed that her nodules had diminished and there was no further recurrence. We have not heard from her since.

48. **A fifty-year-old female** came to the clinic in February 1982 with breast cancer and metastatic lung disease. She had undergone a radical mastectomy, after which dozens of nodes appeared under her arms, across her chest, and over her spine. During radiation her pericardium (the membranous sac enclosing the heart) was burned so severely that she developed pericarditis, necessitating puncturing and draining the pericardium. Chemotherapy had no effect on the growth of her nodules initially. When this patient appeared at the clinic, she carried oxygen and could not walk more than two or three steps without having to stop and use it. We immediately put her on a strong immunization program. We also referred her for modified chemotherapy and additional but minimal radiation. At the time of this writing, scans and echograms indicate she is totally clear. On the morning of her last visit she had jogged two miles on the San Diego beach.

49. **A fifty-seven-year-old female** came to the clinic in October 1978 with cancer of the breast and bone cancer of the left hip. She had had a hysterectomy and an oophorectomy in 1966 and 1967, respectively, before coming to the clinic. We treated her with immunotherapy. A scan in 1979 and another at the end of 1982 showed no evidence of cancer.

50. **A sixty-two-year-old female** came to the clinic in July 1981 after

having had a hysterectomy and mastectomy for adenocarcinoma of the right breast, stage II, followed by chemotherapy. The chemotherapy was too toxic; during this time there was widespread recurrence of nodes with 17 of 26 nodes positive and a large two-inch tumor in her axilla. We treated her with the immunotherapy program. At the time of this writing, recent scans and a physical examination indicate she is clear.

51. **A forty-five-year-old female** came to the clinic in October 1981 with malignant Level III melanoma of the right buttock. After surgical removal and treatment with immunotherapy, she has become completely clear as confirmed by a telephone call to her physician at the time of this writing. She remains on the prevention program.

52. **A sixty-three-year-old female** came to the clinic in December

---

NEWS UPDATE: STUDY FINDS CANCER-RESISTANT COMPOUNDS IN ASPARAGUS

Researchers at Rutgers School of Environmental and Biological Sciences (formerly known as Cook College) led by Dr. Chee-Kok Chin, reported that they had identified a compound in asparagus called "saponin" that prevents leukemia cells from multiplying in lab tests. This finding reported in *Planta Medica* (1997) corroborates similar reports from the National Cancer Institute (NCI) and the Cancer Institute of New Jersey.

Dr. Chin's laboratory found two compounds in asparagus, protodioscin and rutin, that have chemoprotective power against leukemia cells. It appears the protodioscin, a class of compounds called saponins, inhibits the reproduction of a certain leukemia cell line called HL-60. When Dr. Chin submitted protodioscin to the NCI for evaluation, the NCI results showed that "protodioscin has significant inhibitory activity against three panels of cancer cell lines: leukemia, colon cancer, and melanoma."

Further, several reports in China have been attributing antitumor benefits to asparagus. One drug, called *xinxuekang* in Chinese, or XXK, is extracted from a wild yam and uses protodioscin as its active ingredient. It was developed by the Institute of Botany at the Chinese Academy of Sciences and, according to the *NOST China News* (April 19, 2012), is now marketed commercially in Europe by a company named Di'ao, a spinoff of the institute. Available in capsule form, the product recently received approval as a therapeutic medicine by Medicines Evaluation Board of the Netherlands, which opened up the European market.

Of course, the new information about the cancer-resistant compounds in asparagus has given rise to a wave of "miracle" supplements and the usual "miraculous," if anecdotal, case histories. Also, articles have appeared in nutrition journals and periodicals authored by "experts" who claim "scientific evidence" that this or that powder or juice will make your cancer go away. The Internet is full of "asparagus-therapy" stories.

One Internet writer, who calls himself a biochemist but who doesn't identify himself or his credentials, cited a dentist who allegedly discovered that asparagus "might cure cancer." (How a dentist made a dramatic discovery in cancer research is another story entirely.) However, there is no biographical information available on the dentist, no published papers, and no other mention of his name in any clinical trials or university bibliographies.

Anyway, this "biochemist" claims that an "almost hopeless" case of Hodgkin's disease was cured within a year by ingesting daily gobs of pureed asparagus; that a 68-year-old man's bladder tumor disappeared in three months; that a lung cancer patient declared inoperable was back to work five months later; and that a woman was cured of kidney disease and skin cancer after starting asparagus therapy. All investigations of these and similar asparagus-doing cancer cures have resulted in the same conclusion: Hoax!

Once again, these miracles are strictly anecdotal, yet Dr. Chin's scientific research cited above demonstrates that adding asparagus, along with lots of cruciferous veggies, to your diet is the best way to upregulate the chemoprotectors in your immune system.

1981 after a left radical mastectomy, including removal of six positive nodes. We put her on prevention therapy, and she has recently developed small nodes under her scar. She is still on the program. An x-ray in November 1982 revealed no metastasis. In February 1983 her lumps were diminishing. When we called, she was clear.

53. **A fifty-five-year-old female** came to the clinic in November 1981. She was diagnosed as having a 2.5 by 2.8 cm (0.9 by 1.1 in) tumor of the left lung, lower lobe, which was metastatic to five of seven nodes in the area. The September before she came to the clinic, the lobe was removed. A body scan showed bones, liver, and spleen in good condition. The patient had never smoked but had been around heavy smokers all her life. She had neither radiation nor chemotherapy. In February 1982 a chest x-ray showed no pleural effusion (lungs). She is currently following the program, and a recent chest x-ray at the time of this writing showed no evidence of recurrence.

54. **A sixty-two-year-old female** came to the clinic in October 1981 having been declared "terminal" by her physician with cancer of the colon and an extremely large metastasis to her liver. She also had heart problems. She stayed alive for a full year on our program of immunotherapy, but we suddenly lost contact with her at the end of 1982. She is presumed dead.

55. **A sixty-six-year-old female** came to the clinic in June 1981 with cancer of both breasts with metastasis to the ribs. Radiation had no effect but to break down the skin on the wall of her chest. We put her on full immunotherapy. At the end of 1982, echograms, x-rays, and scans showed marked improvement. Only one bad spot in the rib remained. When we called, she was clear.

56. **A sixty-four-year-old male** physician came to the clinic in January 1980 with cancer of the prostate and basal cell cancer of the face. This patient refused radiation or chemotherapy and

was concerned because several members of his family had died of cancer. We put him on the regular program, and tests in January of 1982 indicated he was clear of cancer. A telephone check at the time of this writing confirmed he is still clear. (I also asked this physician for permission to use his name for an expanded case history, but again was refused—EGA.)

57. **A fifty-five-year-old female** came to the clinic in September 1976 after a hysterectomy and with metastasis to the pelvis. She had refused surgery. Chemotherapy resulted in no improvement. After radiation made her severely sick, she terminated both treatments and came to us with a recurrent inoperable mass in her rectum. At the clinic we discovered an inoperable 12 by 12 cm (4.7 by 4.7 in) tumor between her vagina and rectum. At the time of this writing, after almost seven years, she is greatly improved, but not completely well, and remains under treatment. The mass has been reduced to one-fourth its former size. She seems to be progressing, albeit slowly, and is living a normal life.

58. **A seventy-year-old male** came to the clinic in January 1981 with oat-cell cancer of the lung and right neck metastasis. He responded well to immunotherapy. He contacted us in February 1982 and said he was doing well and that his doctors couldn't believe his improvement. This man subsequently died, but there is little doubt that our program prolonged his life at least an additional year.

59. **A twenty-six-year-old female** came to the clinic in June 1981 with a malignant melanoma of the forehead that spread to the right lung and bones. She had had extensive chemotherapy and radiation and went on and off our immunotherapy program at the clinic, never remaining with any one therapy for any length of time. She died in 1982.

60. **A sixty-six-year-old female** came to the clinic in August 1978

with a lymphoma of the small bowel with metastases to the spleen and aorta. She was declared inoperable and "terminal" by her physician after she failed to respond to radiation. We began strong immunotherapy. After the patient started to respond, she moved from New York City to San Diego to be close to the clinic. Scans, ultrasound, and blood chemistries at the time of this writing indicate that she is completely clear of cancer and leading a normal life.

61. **A sixty-year-old female** came to the clinic in April 1982. In 1980 she had had a radical mastectomy with nearly all nodes (thirty-one of thirty-two) positive and was treated with chemotherapy. She had also had cancer of the ribs and sternum treated with 3,000 rads of radiation in July and September 1981. The front of her right breast was inflamed. As we treated her, she improved. In October 1982 her bone scan was negative, and she went home. Unfortunately, she reactivated and came back in poor condition. She started on the program again, and improved. However, she went on and off our program, and eventually died.

62. **A forty-seven-year-old female** came to the clinic in November 1979 with cancer of the breast with metastases to the scapula and adrenals, a mass in her uterus, and infiltration in both lungs. She had had a mastectomy in 1972, an oophorectomy, and then an adrenalectomy (removal of the adrenal glands) in 1979, and several courses of chemotherapy. When she appeared at the clinic she had developed lesions on her pelvis. We treated her with the usual immunotherapy. In 1982 ultrasound showed her lesions diminishing and her chest clear. A telephone check at the time of this writing indicates she is completely clear and feeling fine.

An Invitation Repeatedly Refused

After publishing these findings, and each time she discussed them thereafter, Dr. Virginia always volunteered to provide the patient's medical records to any licensed physician or otherwise qualified researcher (provided the patient gave his or her permission). She also offered to put such researchers or medical examiners in direct touch with the patient and the patient's physician for personal interviewing. She also offered to open her clinic for inspection or educational visits by any physician, organization, or representative of an accredited institution.

Specifically, Dr. Virginia never missed an opportunity in public or private to invite the American Cancer Society and the National Cancer Institute to visit the clinic and make a thorough investigation of her program, her treatments, and her results.

To my knowledge or that of anyone at the clinic, none of her critics ever took her up on it. This fact has always astonished me.

As mentioned earlier, the closest Dr. Virginia's clinic came to professional investigation was an April 15, 1991, issue of the prestigious *New England Journal of Medicine* (*NEJM*), which printed a "Special Article" entitled, "Survival and Quality of Life Among Patients Receiving Unproven as Compared with Conventional Therapy." The "unproven" in the title referred to the Livingston-Wheeler Medical Clinic, and the study compared two sets of 78 patients matched by sex, race, age, diagnosis, and time from the diagnosis of metastatic or recurrent disease, who were enrolled over a period of three years.

The article concluded that there was no difference between the two groups in length of survival. It was published almost a year after her death in June 1990, and there is no record today of who actually provided the *NEJM* investigators with the list of her patients. Her proponents and colleagues at the clinic claimed the study was flawed because it didn't take into account that all her patients had been declared terminal when they appeared at her door.

The *NEJM* article notwithstanding, any official investigator could have walked through her front doors and publicly discredited Dr. Virginia and her theories, yet they chose time after time to criticize her only from afar.

7

Views on Orthodoxy

At this point in Dr. Virginia's story, a review of her thoughts on orthodox treatments (at the time) is in order. A common fallacy committed by her critics, then and now, is the charge that she gave no credit to what are commonly known as the three orthodox cancer treatments. These critics seem to ignore the fact that Dr. Virginia *insisted* that her patients be under an oncologist's care (albeit, as I've said, many of her patients had been declared "terminal" and came to the clinic as a last resort).

The orthodox treatments include:

- Surgery: Cutting out the tumor and hoping it won't grow back or pop up somewhere else.

- Radiation: Destroying the tumor with sharply focused high doses of radiation, and hoping the patient's surrounding vital tissues aren't destroyed in the process.

- Chemotherapy: Introducing certain highly toxic chemicals into the patient's system and hoping they'll attack the tumor and kill it before they kill the patient.

In truth, as we've seen in the previous chapter, Dr. Virginia gave each treatment its due, ascribing to each the level of efficacy she deemed applicable. What she did *not* do was give any of the orthodox treatments credit for cancer remissions.

The White Hats Versus the Black Hats

Dr. Virginia frequently applied the old joke about good news and bad news to the disease of cancer. She told her patients that the good news was that in most cases cancer victims could strengthen their immune systems and recover completely. She thought that, just as with smallpox, tuberculosis, and polio, there was an appropriate immunotherapy protocol that could save the victim's life.

The bad news, she insisted, was that cancer patients would probably be talked into undergoing one of the three orthodox treatments *before* their immune systems were strengthened, and before they eventually realized that those treatments frequently could be more deadly than the disease itself. She argued that each of them, to one degree or another, is aimed at the destruction of the cancer *cell* (along with surrounding healthy cells) and not to the cancer *cause*. In other words, each of the treatments, she said, attacks the manifestation of the disease without working to prevent it. In one lecture, she said it was a lot like shooting mad dogs while ignoring the cure for rabies.

Dr. Virginia considered the orthodox treatments to be drastic measures necessitated by drastic situations. Even though they each offer a certain degree of hope to a desperate patient, they also set up terrible anxieties, and she considered those anxieties justified. (See "Taking Charge: Prostate Surgery or Not?" page 83, for lessons learned by one cancer survivor's mistakes.) While there were—and are—statistics that show how each of these treatments has achieved some measure of remission (she never used the word *cure* in connection with them), each of them also suppresses the immune system's ability to function properly in the life or death battle against the disease. Each of the treatments also reduces the patient's ability or desire to eat, thereby undermining the nutritional requirements in arming the immune system for a long, drawn-out battle.

She considered the whole process a vicious circle that could be, and most frequently was, fatal to the patient. She mocked that other old saw: "The operation was a success, but the patient died." She often considered the so-called orthodox treatments to be worse than the disease itself, with patients dying from them and not from the cancer, and she was fond of saying that her patients' names "were in the phone book, while conventionally treated patients' names were on gravestones."

She posited that radiation and chemotherapy treatments harm the immune system, which needs nutrients to fight back. Yet the treatments usually leave the patient with a lack of appetite, ruining the immune system further, and requiring more treatments, and so on, until the cancer eventually wins the fight. Further, she argued, even while the immune system is being starved of nutrients, the chemicals from chemotherapy, the tissue destruction from radiation, and the trauma of surgery are all keeping the immune system from fighting the cancer cells off, just as if some traitorous munitions maker had outfitted the "good guys" with blank ammunition before they went into battle. The black hats win, because the white hats had no reinforcements. (Dr. Virginia used military analogies often, and very effectively, when explaining the role of the immune system in preventing and fighting cancer. After researching dozens of volumes about how the immune system works, I adopted her and others' military metaphors and wrote the description of the immune system's mechanics described in the next chapter, and she reviewed it, annotated it, and finally approved it.)

One citation Dr. Virginia often gave was that of Richard O. Brennan, M.D., medical director of the Bellevue Metabolic Clinic of Houston and founder of the International Academy of Preventive Medicine. As long ago as 1979, in his book *Coronary? Cancer? God's Answer: Prevent It!* Dr. Brennan wrote:

> Our cancer research is misdirected, inefficient, and inadequate. We have almost as many people living off the disease as are dying from it. The government spends billions on cancer research but at the same time allows known carcinogens in our processed foods;

subsidizes cigarettes; and continues to develop new radiation, surgical, and chemotherapy techniques, when burning, cutting, and
poisoning have already proved largely unsuccessful. Physicians
have not been trained in preventive medicine and, not having experience or knowledge of preventive medicine, they continue the out-
moded but orthodox approach of treating symptoms rather than
the entire body.

The charge against cigarettes has changed since Dr. Brennan's
book, and certain advice in preventive medicine—such as diet—is
currently growing in popularity, but Dr. Virginia's general attitude
was pretty well summed up by that passage.

Dr. Virginia contended that if you asked an honest oncologist for
the truth, he would tell you that no more than 15 or 20 percent of
patients derived any benefit from his treatments. Such inflamma-
tory statements, which Dr. Virginia was wont to make at the drop
of a hat, inevitably backed her against the wall. When I asked her
what specifically she had against the orthodox treatments, she gave
the following explanations. These were essentially her explanations
to cancer patients about what they could expect from orthodox treatments (and in many cases, her patients had already validated her
opinion).

Surgery

Dr. Virginia always stated upfront that surgery had a definite place
in the immunotherapy approach to cancer treatment. She recommended it frequently at her clinic because, whenever possible, it
was best to remove large masses of tumor cells from the patient
(she called it "debulking") in order to give the immune system
some relief in its comeback fight against the disease. She considered that when a tumor of billions of cells multiplying fright-
fully fast was present, she would be asking a lot of the patient's
immune system to catch up when she began her immunotherapy.
In other words, she was in agreement that removing the tumor

mass by surgical means was cutting down the number of guys in black hats.

But she claimed that most surgeons and cancer physicians don't understand that cancer is a *systemic* disease. The tumor was only a symptom of the disease, she said; the disease causes the tumor, and not vice versa. Frequently when a surgeon has removed a large mass and made a wide dissection, he will comment that he "got it all." This is supposed to be good news, but in the majority of cases, even today, nothing is done to raise the patient's immunity. Also in the majority of cases, there is a recurrence of the cancer within months or a few years.

So Dr. Virginia often considered surgery to be a legitimate first line of defense in postponing the deadly growth of more cancer cells, but she worried that the traumatic effects of surgery would also postpone the patient's recovery. Chances of recovery, she figured, were worsened by the fact that even after surgery, the patient would still have the disease, at least until the patient's immune system was fortified to the maximum level of strength.

In many cases, however, Dr. Virginia achieved great success in beginning immunotherapy treatments immediately and continuing them until the patient's own immune system killed off the tumor. In most of such cases, the cancer was detected early, and before the patient had been subjected to radiation or chemotherapy.

Radiation

In the early days, this treatment method was thought to be a great boon to medicine. Then, as better equipment was developed, specialists theorized that radiating the entire body would destroy the seeds of cancer. Today, radiation is still held in high regard, and Dr. Virginia conceded that radiating a person at a single point, with a single sharply focused beam, could help a patient *in one specific spot*. But she considered it dangerous. Ever since the bombings of Hiroshima and Nagasaki in August of 1945, cancer researchers have become convinced of one unalterable fact: radiation destroys human tissue. Not only that, but radiation destroys human tissue *forever*.

Dr. Virginia pointed to the headlines to make her point. Nuclear plants malfunction and the incidence of cancer increases in the immediate community. Radiation exposure during nuclear tests in the Pacific led to increased bone and other cancers in veterans decades later. Even diagnostic x-rays, considered an innocuous tool of doctors the world over, has come under cancer-causing scrutiny. Therefore, she concluded, did it make sense to radiate a person who already had cancer?

Because the body is a compact system, it is difficult to radiate a single spot without radiating surrounding healthy tissue. If the rectum or colon is radiated, a lot of the lower bowel is also radiated. If the lung is radiated, so will be the ribs, the trachea, the esophagus, the bronchia. Radiation wasn't then, and isn't today, a simple procedure, and its success rate is still quite low.

A patient's immune system is drastically compromised by radiation. The proof that this is true is simple: in organ transplant surgery, the procedure is accompanied by a combination of radiation and chemotherapy to *weaken* the patient's immune system, so that the organ will not be rejected.

Chemotherapy

Dr. Virginia's wrath was especially acute when aimed at this form of treatment. She considered the drugs and chemicals used in chemotherapy to be so toxic, so powerfully destructive to tumors, that they were bound to destroy a patient's immune system as well—thereby canceling any positive effects the treatment may have. She was fond of quoting another physician who once said, "Chemicals and drugs make a battlefield of your body—and when was the last time you saw anything beautiful growing on a battlefield?"

Chemotherapy is necessarily a systemic treatment, she argued, hence the toxicity of the chemotherapeutic agents is spread throughout the patient's entire body. She claimed that no physician or specialist could determine beforehand what a patient's reaction to chemotherapy would be, and she was a vocal advocate of increased research to determine the ability of patients to be immunized against chemical agents.

Taking Charge I: Prostate Surgery or Not?

Virgil E. B. Lawrence is perhaps the foremost lay authority west of the Mississippi on prostate cancer and its treatment. He is a thirty-year survivor of prostate cancer (PCa) and a self-made expert on this condition. Because of his tedious research over the years, he wants to caution male readers against making big mistakes after their first PCa diagnosis.

He writes:

In 1986 I had suddenly began experiencing acute pains in my kidney area and decided to go directly to a urologist. I was forty-nine years old. He gave me a digital rectal exam to palpate my prostate and ordered a prostate-specific antigen (PSA) blood test. My PSA was 14.0, which warranted further testing. A computed tomography (CT) scan was done to see if there were any "surprises," and the internal organs looked normal. A bone scan was done to see if the cancer had spread to the bones, and the results came back negative. However—and this is a very important "however"—it was most likely a *false* negative. Meaning that while the test did not detect cancer in the bones, it was there nevertheless! It turns out a bone scan is not sensitive enough to detect small amounts of cancer, and PCa usually spreads to the bones after it escapes from the prostate.

Now, having said all this, here were my mistakes:

MISTAKE 1: Following my urologist's advice to have surgery. Like many men, I readily agreed to have my prostate removed out of fear. I just wanted the cancer *out!* No second opinion, no research, no self-education—just fear-driven compliance with the MD's recommendation. A urologist may frighten the patient into submitting to a radical prostatectomy (removal of the prostate). If the patient tells his urologist that he wants to seek other opinions or to get more educated about PCa, the usual response of "OK, but don't wait too long" can have a subliminal message that quick action is required, when it actually isn't.

Over the years, and having talked to hundreds of patients I have learned that the best course of action would have been to get out of the urologist's office and locate a medical oncologist. After a prostate cancer diagnosis, a patient should get educated by talking to friends, relatives and neighbors, attending support groups, viewing videos, and talking to others who have had a similar experience. Do *not* rush into a treatment before examining all your options. Many physicians believe, and I agree, that PCa is a systemic disease; hence, local treatments like surgery, radiation (see next!), cryosurgery, and seed implants are useless.

MISTAKE 2: Following my urologist's advice to have radiation treatments. After the surgery, I foolishly submitted to external beam radiation therapy (high-dose radiation) to the pelvic area. This was supposedly to "clean up any residual cancer cells left behind," because malignant cells were found in some of the lymph nodes that were removed during the procedure. Eight months after the radiation, I had sharp, stinging pains in my back. A follow-up scan showed the cancer had metastasized to the spine and ribs. The urologist now suggested I take diethylstilbestrol (DES), a synthetic female hormone that is known to cause strokes and heart attacks. By this time I was, in fact, doing my homework and I refused the DES because I knew of its dangers.

How did I cure the cancer after it had spread to my bones? (I am not afraid to use the word "cure.") I had read of a PCa treatment called combinational hormone blockade (CHB), a treatment modality the FDA approved in March 1989 that combines two drugs that essentially cut off the cancer cells' "food" and block replacement nutrients. (At the time there were only three oncologists in California who were using it.) The first drug is either leuprolide (Lupron) or goserelin (Zoledex), which brings down the testosterone level to the "castration level." In short, it enables you to avoid an orchiectomy and keep your testicles. But the adrenal glands can still produce androgens (male hormones), which can be converted to dihydrotestosterone (DHT), which in turn will continue to feed the malignant cells. Therefore, the second drug, flutamide (Eulexin), blocks the uptake of the DHT into the malignant cells, which kills them. They literally starve to death. In a five-year study at MD Anderson Hospital in Houston and reported in *Clinical Oncology Alert* (1997), only 15 percent of patients survived when treated by radiation alone. But a whopping 85 percent survived when the radiation was supplemented with CHB.

Within six months after starting CHB therapy, the two lesions on my bones were undetectable by a bone scan. My PSA went to less than 0.1 and has remained there ever since. In August 1997, I learned that long-term deprivation of testosterone leads to osteoporosis, so I voluntarily went off the CHB against the advice of my oncologist. (For tips on how to argue with your doctor, read Dr. Bernie Segal's *Love, Medicine, and Miracles*, 1986.)

MISTAKE 3: Not seeking more quickly a medical oncologist who is familiar with alternative treatments. Robert Leibowitz is a medical oncologist in Los Angeles who prescribes triple androgen blockade (TAB). This protocol adds a third drug to CHB: finasteride (Proscar) or dustasteride (Avodart). Proscar or Avodart are also used to block the production of DHT, which is five times more likely than testosterone to feed the cancer cells. Many medical doctors will claim that the TAB treatment has not yet been proven. Yet, Charles Huggins, who won the Nobel Prize in Medicine in 1966, published two related papers as far back as 1941. To read about his work, see Stephen Strum's article in the archives of *PCRI Insights* (October 2000), a publication of the Prostate Cancer Research Institute, entitled "Intermittent Hormonal Deprivation." Go to the second part of the article, "Understanding the Endocrinology of Prostate Cancer."

I am convinced that surgery and radiation should be the *last* resort of the PCa patient. I'm angry with myself for allowing my prostate to be surgically removed. I urge all men with a PCa diagnosis to contact Patient Advocates for Advanced Cancer Treatments (PAACT), an organization that encourages men with prostate cancer to take charge of their bodies and their treatments before making a major decision that will affect their quality of life and sex life. After surgery, a urologist will attempt to correct your sexual ability with hormone shots or penile implants. (Erectile dysfunction is a one of two main complications from radical prostatectomy; the other is urinary incontinence.) I suffered from both. Why subject yourself to such treatments? Hormonal blockade is a much safer path to preserve a man's sexual function.

Consider this: 40 percent of all men over 40 have evidence of PCa. Only 7 to 8 percent will have symptoms needing treatment, and then only 2 to 3 percent will die of the disease. Autopsies are showing that most men over 50 have some form of PCa when they die. If only 3 percent die from PCa that means 97 percent died *with* it! If only 7 to 8 percent need treatment, that means that 9 out of 10 men don't. Most forms of PCa are slow growing. Take your time, be open, and consider all your options.

Indeed, as Mr. Lawrence points out, it's because PCa is a slow-growing cancer that newly diagnosed men should realize that they have a lot of time to do a thorough search of every possible treatment alternative. Dr. Virginia did not prescribe chemotherapy or radiation for her PCa patients—both for that reason and because there are so many other promising treatments being developed. As stated elsewhere, her use of BCG, while ridiculed 25 years ago, is now the preferred initial treatment for bladder cancer, and BCG is being used widely in the treatment of prostate cancer.

Self-Defeating Treatments

Did Dr. Virginia have anything *good* to say about orthodox treatments? Only these two things in general:

1. Each can be temporarily useful in *most* cases, and more effective in *some* cases. Surgery can remove *some* tumors; radiation and chemotherapy can diminish *some* tumors.

2. The effectiveness of each orthodox treatment can be enhanced by an accompanying program of nutritional support to boost the patient's immune system. (I once spoke with a San Diego oncologist, who refused to be identified in print, who said that those of his patients who had already been put on a sound nutritional and immunological regimen at Dr. Virginia's clinic had an "exceptionally" higher rate of recovery than his other patients.)

In a nutshell, Dr. Virginia considered surgery, radiation, and chemotherapy to be ultimately self-defeating. That is, they suppressed the immune system while trying to fortify it. What's more, all too frequently the patient's immune system is so compromised that other infections are contracted, ultimately leading to the patient's death even before the cancer itself kills him (as in pneumonia, for example).

She claimed that the reason these orthodox treatments were still used despite the growing knowledge of the immune system's role, was that there was a great deal of political pressure within the medical establishment against innovators. She was fond of reciting a litany of far-thinking, innovative, intuitive scientists whose research investigations and clinical discoveries leap-frogged ahead of conventional thinking, but who were castigated and ostracized for daring to present their theories. Copernicus and Galileo were threatened with imprisonment and torture unless they recanted their theories about Earth's position in the universe. A simple country doctor named Edward Jenner observed that milkmaids who contracted cowpox were somehow immunized against smallpox. When he vaccinated some of his young patients with a cowpox vaccine, and they didn't get smallpox, Jenner was attacked by the medical authorities because he couldn't explain *why* his vaccine worked. Jenner is today considered the father of immunology.

Louis Pasteur, who refined Jenner's work with his anthrax and rabies vaccines, and who actually brought the new science of immunization to the world at large, was ridiculed for most of his life for his assertion that there were infectious "microbes" and other organisms that couldn't be seen with the naked eye. After all, he was a chemist—not a doctor! And Dr. Virginia would never fail to mention that it took more than 400 years to convince surgeons to wash their hands before entering the operating room.

Certainly, as we'll see in later pages, there are similar pioneers alive today, working at the cutting edge of medical innovation and scientific discovery. Since Dr. Virginia's death many of them are gaining an increasing voice in the medical establishment, which seems lately to be ever so slightly willing to listen to new theories. But when Dr. Virginia used the words "nutrition," "bacteria," and "vaccine" in connection with the prevention and treatment of cancer, medical establishmentarians winced and turned their collective head away from such "quackery." She dismissed such rejection with one of her favorite sayings, "Doctors are always down on something they're not up on."

8

How Your Immune System Works

Your immune system is your defense force: the total protection your body offers against foreign invaders that would contaminate, or infect, your body. The cliché in medicine is to compare the immune system and these "invaders" to military action, with armies, reinforcements, and various weaponry. However, it has become a cliché only because it is an accurate analogy and approximates the drama of immune reaction in the body. Your body does, in fact, employ a patrol force, a strike force, a counter-attacking army with reinforcements, and even bombs and undercover spies who "mark" the enemy invaders as targets for attack.

The immune system, though complex and designed with redundant backup systems that by comparison would make any sophisticated aerospace computer look as simple as a light switch, is your *only* protection against innumerable afflictions and diseases. It destroys literally thousands of *potentially* disease-causing substances in your body, as well as those substances that we know are disease-causing. It also participates in the repair and healing process after an affliction has been eradicated. This heroic immune system protects your body both from within (against the byproducts of your biochemical reactions) and from without (against pollutants, poisons, etc., and from *all* foreign substances and toxic agents, including bacteria, viruses, and chemicals). It can discriminate between what is part of your body and what is not; between what is friendly and what is enemy; between what wants to help you and what wants to kill you. If you did not have an immune system, you would die within weeks or else spend your life in a hermetically sealed plastic bubble.

Perhaps as you are reading this book you have been reminded of the statement: "We all have cancer in our bodies; it's just that our immune system is keeping it in check." If you were to change the statement to: "We all have cancer-causing *bugs* in our bodies," it would be absolutely true. It is our immune system that is keeping us from developing cancer, and it is the breakdown of our immune system that allows cancer to grow.

The quality of your health, both physical and mental, is a good way to measure how strong your immune system is in general. Do you get colds? (Don't say "everyone does"—many people don't, and it's no accident.) Do you catch every flu bug that comes around? Do you smoke? Do you drink too much? (Don't analyze your social group—people know deep in their hearts whether they do or not.) Is your diet one of junk foods, frozen and processed foods, meat and poultry, high in sugar and devoid of vitamin and mineral supplements? If the answer to these questions is yes, then your immune system is not at its peak strength.

If, on the other hand, you never get sick; if you can visit sick friends and not catch their colds or flus; if you don't smoke; if you drink only moderately; if your diet is high in raw vegetables and low in meat, poultry, and junk foods; and if you have a substantial vitamin supplement program high in vitamins A, C, D, and E, then you may be sure your immune system is working at a high-strength level.

The reason, then, that you get sick is that your immune system is weak. (As always, remember, there are exceptions—an especially virulent bug might attack an immunologically strong person and lay the person low, but the immune system is what will fight it off and have the person back on his or her feet quickly, whereas the immunologically weak person will be sick for a long time, perhaps contract other infections or symptoms, and take a long time to recover.)

A Disease of the Immune System

Cancer is a disease of the immune system. Or, more accurately, it is a disease of a *weak* immune system. Your immunity must drop to a very low level before cancer can grow, and when it drops to an extremely low and weak level the cancer cells start to spread. Your body has no defense against them, or what small defense it has is not enough. The invaders on the beach keep landing more and more troops and marching inland with their machine guns to capture the territory, while your pitifully small and poorly armed resistance force can do nothing to stop the enemy's progress.

Every cancer patient who came to Dr. Virginia's clinic had a severely depressed immune system.

It follows, then, that if you maintain a strong and healthy immune system, your resistance to cancer will be high. And the ability of your immune system to successfully prevent cancer is dependent to a large degree on your state of nutrition. If your diet provides all the nutrients needed by your immune system to maintain maximum strength, and if your liver and other organs are producing the proper amounts of enzymes to process these nutrients, the chances are much higher than average that you will not contract cancer. Little did Dr. Virginia expect to find, in her early days of research, that the shortage of a single vitamin or mineral would have drastic effects on immunity. But experiment after experiment, test after test, has shown this to be true. Conversely, *increased* amounts of certain vitamins and minerals can strengthen your resistance to infection and disease.

This is where she got into trouble with the medical profession. There was then, but not so much today, almost always a knee-jerk reaction to vitamins and minerals—against the one who is proposing them—on the part of American physicians. Even though the aforementioned 1997 study, referred to in Chapter 2, authorized by the National Academy of Sciences concluded that we should eat more foods high in certain vitamins to avoid cancer (they stopped short of recommending supplements), the average doctor winced when any disease therapy included a dietary regimen and vitamin supplements. Today, most physicians acknowledge that vitamins can be an important part of maintaining a robust immune system. But there is still disagreement in some circles. TV personality and author Mehmet Oz, M.D., takes a daily multivitamin and extra vitamin D, and so does celebrated nutrition guru Andrew Weil, M.D. But nationally syndicated radio host Dean Edell, M.D., (now retired) almost daily warned his listeners that vitamins are a waste of money. (See "News Update: The Good News about Vitamin D," below.)

Dr. Virginia recommended a lot of vitamin A analogs in her dietary regimen, for both the pre-cancer and post-cancer programs, yet doctors still today warn their patients that too much vitamin A is toxic. A person taking 10,000 international units (IU) per day is

---

NEWS UPDATE:
THE GOOD NEWS ABOUT VITAMIN D

There is such a large body of research regarding the role of vitamin D in the prevention of carcinogenesis that today it is generally accepted in medical circles that vitamin D deficiency can cause cancers of the prostate, breast, uterus, and colon, among others. Conversely, supplementing one's diet with vitamin D can greatly lower the risk of cancer.

Research shows that we don't get enough vitamin D in our diets. In the March 2007 editorial written for the *American Journal of Clinical Nutrition*, University of Toronto professor and vitamin-D scientist Dr. Reinhold Vieth stated, "Geography, season, skin color, and sun-related behavior are the main predictors of vitamin D nutritional status. Correction of low (vitamin D) concentrations can happen only if some or all of the following are implemented: the encouragement of safe, moderate exposure of skin to ultraviolet light, appropriate increases in food fortification with vitamin D, and the provision of higher doses of vitamin D in supplements for adults."

The current daily adult recommendation for vitamin D is 200–600 international units (IU). However, Dr. Bruce H. Hollis, a biochemist at the Medical University of South Carolina, said in the *Journal of Nutrition* (2005), that the recommendation is "very inadequate when one considers that a 10–15 minute whole-body exposure to peak summer sun will generate and release up to 20,000 IU of vitamin D_3 into the circulation."

One seldom hears physicians recommend dietary supplements of any kind; they usually stress a "balanced diet" instead. So it is rare indeed that such a large body of physicians today recommends supplemental vitamin D.

Vitamin D is technically not a vitamin. It is a group of fat-soluble hormone-like nutrients. Vitamin D has two forms: vitamin D_2, which is made by plants, and vitamin D_3, which is made naturally by the body when the skin is exposed to ultraviolet radiation in sunlight. There are 3,000 studies currently being conducted on vitamin D's role in cancer prevention. Some highlights include:

- Protects against cancer: In the 1970s, the first sunlight exposure vs. vitamin D results came from epidemiologic studies known as geographic correlation studies. In these studies, an inverse relationship was found between sunlight exposure levels in a given geographic area and the rates of incidence and death for certain cancers in that area. Individuals living in southern latitudes were found to have lower rates of incidence and death for these cancers than those living at northern latitudes. Because sunlight/ultraviolet (UV) exposure is necessary for the production of vitamin D_3, researchers hypothesized that variation in vitamin D levels accounted for the observed relationships.

   In 2011, Dr. Cedric Garland, widely regarded as the foremost authority on vitamin D and an epidemiologist at the University of California, San Diego (UCSD), showed that colorectal cancer incidence in the United States is dramatically high in the Northeast and lowest in the South and Southwest. This, he explained, is because the Northeast has a thicker ozone layer, concentrated pollutants from combustion, and a colder climate with less sunlight on average than the rest of the country.

- Reduces cancer deaths: Several epidemiologic studies have reported an association between vitamin D and reduced mortality from specific cancers, such as colorectal, breast, and prostate. In 2007, Dr. D. Michal Freedman and his coworkers at the National Cancer Institute reported in its journal that among the 16,818 participants in the Third National Health and Nutrition Examination Survey, those with high vitamin D blood levels (above 80 nanograms per milliliter [ng/mL]) had a 72 percent lower risk of colorectal cancer death than those with lower vitamin D blood levels (less than 50 ng/mL).

- Lowers cancer risk: Also in 2007, the *American Journal of Clinical Nutrition* reported on a team of researchers led by Dr. Joan Lappe from the Osteoporosis Research Center at Creighton University in Omaha, Nebraska, who studied 1,179 healthy, postmenopausal women, fifty-five years or older and cancer free for at least ten years. The subjects were randomly assigned to take daily dosages of either 1,400–1,500 mg of supplemental calcium, 1,400–1,500 mg supplemental calcium plus 1,100 IU of vitamin D_3, or a placebo. (Vitamin D helps the body absorb and retain calcium.) Over the four-year trial, women in the calcium/vitamin D_3 group experienced a 60 percent or greater reduced risk of cancer than their peers in the placebo group, who were not consuming these supplements.

  Two years later, in the *Annals of Epidemiology*, Garland (aforementioned) and researchers at UCSD's Moores Cancer Center used a complex computer model to predict that intake of vitamin D_3 and calcium would prevent 58,000 new cases of breast cancer and 49,000 new cases of colorectal cancer annually in the North America. The researchers' model also predicted that 75 percent of deaths from these cancers could be prevented with adequate intake of vitamin D_3 and calcium. To prevent vitamin D deprivation, Garland recommended maintaining one's vitamin D serum level at 40–60 ng/mL, and taking vitamin D supplements for those with lower levels.

- Reduces tumor size: A 2010 study by Dr. JoEllen Welsh, a researcher at the State University of New York, Albany, treated human breast cancer samples with a potent form of vitamin D. Within a few days, half the cancer cells shriveled up and died. Welsh said the vitamin has the same effect as tamoxifen (Nolvadex), a drug commonly pre-scribed for breast cancer treatment. "What happens is that vitamin D enters the cells and triggers the cell death process," she told ABC's *Good Morning America.* "It's similar to what we see when we treat cells with Tamoxifen." The vitamin's effects were even more dra-matic on breast cancer cells injected into mice. After several weeks of treatment, the cancer tumors in the mice shrank by an average of more than 50 percent. Some tumors disappeared. Similar results have been achieved on colon and prostate cancer tumors.

- Blocks cancer cell growth: In 2011, as reported in *PLoS One,* Spanish researcher Hector G. Palmer published a paper investigating factors controlling human colon cancer progression. Part of his abstract states: "Vitamin D_3 has antitumor activity in addition to its classical action on calcium metabolism and bone tissue biology. It is thought to regulate the expression of multiple target genes and thus modu-late processes critical for tumor growth and metastases."

   In 2012, a Spanish team of researchers led by Professor Alberto Muñoz at the Institute for Biomedical Research at the School of Med-icine of the Universidad Autónoma de Madrid studied the molecular basis of the protective role that vitamin D exerts against colon can-cer cells. His findings, which appeared in *Endocrine Related Cancer,* are among the first to demonstrate that vitamin D "drastically changes the gene expression of cancer cells, inhibiting proliferation and promoting differentiation."

Recommendations? They vary widely. The U.S. Recommended Dietary Allowance of 400–600 IU daily is generally agreed to be too low. Some sources recommend 1,000 IU, but others are even higher. Dr. Mark Haussler, a researcher and professor at the University of Arizona College of Medicine, cautions "It's certainly not going to be the magic bullet that's going to cure any (diseases), but it will lower the risk. Therefore, I'm a believer in a higher dose [of supplemental vitamin D_3]. Given that it is going to depend on latitude and other things, a good recommendation Is 2,000 IU." The best advice is to have your serum vitamin D tested and then follow the advice of your doctor, who should be up on the latest recommendations.

Clearly, Dr. Virginia's idea of a nutrition-based regimen as an integral part of a multimodal treatment program had a strong molecular basis. She would be very excited about the work of Dr. Garland and others today!

told to be careful and take only 5,000. A person taking 25,000 IU sends the physician into shock. A cancer patient, who needs all the vitamin A possible, is given only token amounts of vitamin supplements. The truth is that a healthy adult can take much more than 5,000 IU a day without experiencing any toxic effects. Remember, my father was dying of cancer of the bladder when his doctor cautioned him against taking too much vitamin C because he "might get kidney stones." The poor man was wasting away and trying to slow down his disease, yet his doctor was worried about an extremely *rare* effect of too much vitamin C! In short, the American Medical Association is still coming out of the Middle Ages on the subject of vitamin supplements. On the other hand, perhaps if patients and lawyers were not so quick to sue for malpractice, or if there were not so much vitamin quackery, we'd have more enlightened attitudes from our family physicians.

The question now arises: Is being "well" simply not being sick, or are there varying levels of "wellness"? Can we be only a "little bit well" (i.e., just barely not sick) "pretty well," and "very, very well"?

The answer is yes. A person can be only well enough so as not to be sick, or can be extremely well so as to feel absolutely great all the time! And the reason is that the strength or weakness of the immune system determines how you feel—whether you're barely well and will get sick at the drop of a hat, or extremely well and seldom get sick.

Immunity and the Diet Connection

Dr. Virginia believed the great changes in American eating patterns over the past several decades were largely responsible for the high rate of cancer. She believed the modern diet is simply deficient in providing the nutrition essentials that maintain a healthy, vital immunity to cancer. Hence, with these lowered defenses, cancer can start and spread with little or no opposition by our bodies. All too often, what we put into or mouths either causes or directly contributes to the onset of cancer through the depression of our immunity.

It is becoming an old story in these enlightened times, and you've heard it before in books, articles, or TV interviews. We won't belabor it here, but to review it quickly: A century ago most Americans ate food grown in their own gardens or farms. They picked ripe fruit from the orchard and ate vegetables fresh from the fields. Their food came directly from the garden to their dinner table—and the field itself was chock full of minerals and excellent nutritive soils. Today, most food comes to us from fields hundreds, even thousands, of miles away. Frequently, it reaches our table only after detouring though factories and processing plants, through complex machines that have been devised to peel, cook, and preserve fresh foods, transforming them into bagged, canned, frozen, or dried products. Fruits and vegetables are sprayed, waxed, pickled, sweetened, dyed, conditioned, and sterilized—and are reduced to only a fraction of the nutrients nature intended by the time we eat them. Every day, Americans consume the contents of more than 90 million cans and jars and more than 40 million pounds of frozen and packaged foods.

While we pride ourselves on being the "best-fed" people in history, our diets *rarely* provide us with all the nutrients needed by our bodies and immune systems. It is perhaps the ultimate irony that we are responsible for crippling our own immune systems through nutritional starvation. The best-fed nation in history also has the highest incidence of cancer and heart disease. What is needed is for everyone to realize that what you eat affects the chances of getting cancer, and that there is a scientifically proven diet that guarantees fortification of the immune system against cancer and other diseases. (See "News Update: Cancer-Fighting and Immune-Boosting Foods," page 100.)

Your Health Bank Account

Let's look at this a different way. Your immune system is like your "health savings account." Deposits are made in currencies of good food, avoidance of toxic substances, and maintenance of a positive mental outlook. If the immune account has grown as a result of healthy deposits, and the time comes for a "withdrawal," your immune forces can be mobilized to combat disease. However, when your account is overdrawn, disease can only gain a foothold. There is no borrowing—your immune system has no credit rating. It is either solvent or broke.

When patients came to the Livingston-Wheeler Clinic, Dr. Virginia tested their "immune financial condition" as quickly and accurately as a banker can check your balance in his computer. Unfortunately, what she found so often in patients with advanced cancer is that their immune systems were bankrupt.

The Immune System

How your body resists infection, how it rallies the various warrior groups to do battle against the toxic enemies that would like to kill you, is one of the most profound miracles of life. The subject is worth an entire book, and indeed an excellent one was written a while back for the layperson that still explains quite well today how your immune system works. I heartily refer you to *The Body Is the Hero* (1976) by Ronald J. Glasser, M.D. Every cancer patient, and indeed everyone interested in personal health and immunity, should read this outstanding book. For our purposes, here, however, I shall simply try to give an overview of what happens when your body fights infection.

Like the army, navy, and air force, there are three important "services" that make up our immune system's defenses: antibodies, granulocytes (white cells), and something with the unusual name of "complement." Let us briefly acquaint ourselves with each system.

Antibodies

The antibody system is the army. An antibody is a protein substance in the blood serum that is produced as a reacting agent to attack and destroy an invading foreign body. The foreign substance that incites the antibody's attack is called an "antigen." This antigen-antibody reaction is generally specific to a certain disease— that is, an antibody will only attack the antigen that instigated its production.

How antibodies work is one of the first miracles of immunity. Each invading body, an attacking microbe, has upon its surface a "marker" which distinguishes it from any other organism, much the same as fingerprints are unique to each individual. These markers are simply molecular configurations of the microbe's membrane. The marker is like the swastika on a World War II German tank or the red ball insignia on the Japanese Zero airplanes. They identified the enemy for our own cannons to shoot at. These markers, which distinguish the antigens, become the identifying insignia for our antibodies to attack. Despite all the dead cells, impurities, broken down bits and pieces of enzymes and hormones, and general microorganic "garbage" continuously flowing through our bloodstream, our plasma cells know what's friendly and harmless and what is a "foreign" body bent on attacking and destroying our tissues.

Newborn babies do not have their own antibodies, and so they use their mothers' to fight early infections. Then as the baby is slowly exposed to germs that may give it scarlet fever, pneumonia, chicken pox, and so on, it creates its own antibodies that attack and neutralize those deadly microbes. When the baby is vaccinated—immunized against specific diseases—it is given an extremely small amount of the antigen disease, thus forming antibodies that attack it and keep the immune system fortified against that specific antigen.

These few indications are merely to show that medical science is finally coming around to acknowledging what Dr. Virginia first proposed half a century ago: that nutrition plays an important role in the *total* cancer-fighting arsenal. There are thousands of studies being conducted around the world that are proving cancer-fighting plant chemicals not only do exist but also that the nearest grocery store may be your cheapest dispensary.

Granulocytes

The second line of defense in our immunization forces is called "granulocytes," or granulated white cells. This is our navy. Whereas the antibodies are our "standing army," ready to be called into action when the invaders launch an attack, the granulocytes are our patrolling PT boats and coast guard cutters, constantly mobile in

---

NEWS UPDATE: CANCER-FIGHTING AND IMMUNE-BOOSTING FOODS

Dr. Virginia's emphasis on nutrition as an essential part of a cancer treatment protocol is just as important as the vaccine itself. Here are a few compounds in foods that have been found to fight cancer and boost the immune system.

CITRUS FRUIT: In its March 2013 *Clinical Summary* update, the Memorial Sloan-Kettering Cancer Center, referencing several published studies in respected medical journals, issued a clinical summary suggesting that the rind of citrus fruits may have important anticancer properties. It cited a substance called "d-limonene," derived from the peels of citrus fruits, as being taken orally by patients to prevent and treat cancer. The center is urging further research "to determine if d-limonene has a role in the prevention and treatment of cancer."

Also in the citrus fruit category, Isaac Eliaz, an Israeli physician and science researcher, has been studying a substance called "pectin," a soluble fiber found in the peel of oranges and lemons. It seems a molecular variant of pectin, called "modified citrus pectin," or MCP, can affect a cancer-cell protein called "galectin-3," a glue-like substance that many studies have shown helps cancer cells clump together, hence promoting growth and metastasis. One such study of melanoma in rats published by *Cancer Microenvironment* in 2008 showed that MCP reduced the spread of cancer by a whopping 90 percent.

FERMENTED WHEAT GERM: A nutritional supplement that has been well researched for cancer patients is a fermented wheat-germ extract developed by Hungarian chemist Máté Hidvégi, based on research initiated many years ago by Dr. Albert Szent-Györgyi, a recipient of the Nobel Prize in Medicine for his discovery of vitamin C. Dr. Szent-Györgyi, who died in 1986 before completing his research, theorized that naturally occurring compounds in wheat germ called quinones could prevent cancer growth.

As the story goes, shortly before Dr. Hidvegi's great discovery was made, his grant ran out and he had no money to continue. He started praying fervently to the Blessed Virgin Mary for a new grant, and the very next day a benefactor appeared and gave him $100,000 to keep working. He subsequently developed a patented process of fermenting wheat germ with baker's yeast, yielding a powerful extract called fermented wheat germ extract. This concentrated extract, called Avemar (from "Ave Maria," in gratitude for the Blessed Virgin's intervention), is now one of the most well-researched natural substances, with more than 100 studies described in over 20 peer-reviewed medical journals. (See Memorial Sloan-Kettering Cancer Center's "Clinical Summary" on Avemar, updated Feb. 19, 2014, with 18 references cited.) Because cancer cells *love* glucose and glucose-providing products, which allow them to proliferate, Avemar—and other concentrated wheat germ extracts—work by inhibiting glucose metabolism in cancer cells, thus "starving" them of the glucose they crave.

POMEGRANATES: Medical researchers have pretty well established that prostate problems are caused not only by lowered levels of testosterone in men, but also by elevated levels of estrogen. This information has triggered several studies that show compounds such as ellagic acid and punicic acid have powerful prostate cancer-fighting properties. And . . . ta-da! . . . these compounds are plentiful in pomegranates!

Dr. Allan Pantuck and his associates at the University of California, Los Angeles, Jonsson Comprehensive Cancer Center studied a group of men with previously treated prostate cancer, giving them an 8-ounce glass of pomegranate juice daily. The results, reported in the July 2006 issue of *Clinical Cancer Research,* indicated that their PSA levels were kept stable. Specifically, they observed an average increase in doubling times (the time it takes for a rising PSA to double) from 15 to 54 months.

A similar University of Quebec 2010 study, published in the *Journal of Agricultural and Food Chemistry,* found that punicic acid in pomegranates inhibited prostate cell growth. In yet another study, pomegranate juice significantly extended the time for PSA levels to double in men who had undergone previous treatment for prostate cancer. At the University of California, Riverside, researchers also reported that phytochemicals in pomegranates had beneficial prostate cancer effects (*UCR Today,* 2010).

SHIITAKE MUSHROOMS: The Chinese have been using mushrooms in medical treatment for thousands of years, but recently medical journals have been reporting that extracts from shiitake mushrooms have cancer-fighting properties. The first human beta-glucan trial was in 1975 when Dr. Peter Mansell of the National Cancer Institute injected it into the malignant skin cancer nodules of nine patients and, as he reported in the *Journal of the National Cancer Institute,* the nodules were "strikingly reduced in as short a period as five days" and some smaller lesions had completely disappeared.

A substance in the mushroom called lentinan is the hero. The Memorial Sloan-Kettering Cancer Center issued a medical bulletin in August 2013 explaining that lentinan has a molecule called beta-glucan that may reduce tumor size and kill cancer cells altogether. It cited referenced scientific papers with encouraging results in carcinomas, and colorectal and pancreatic cancers. As always, it seems, these reports end with "studies are needed," but organic mushroom extracts are available containing large quantities of lentinan.

our bloodstreams, searching the channels of our bodies for any signs of poisonous material that would do us harm. When this search-and-destroy force does find an invader, it mobilizes millions of troops to attack it relentlessly until it has been destroyed. These white cells are in a constant battle deep inside the bloodstream constantly trying to engulf bacteria and destroy them, while the bacteria themselves are constantly emitting their poisons and trying, in turn, to kill our strike forces.

If you were to put a group of granulocytes in a dish of salt water, you would see them casually swimming around, as gracefully as you please, seemingly with no destination and at complete ease. But when you introduce a single bacterium into that tranquil scene, the drama begins as if a starting gun had been sounded. The granulocytes stop, as if alerted by a silent alarm signal to impending danger, and then they begin to prowl through the water, looking for something. Finally they spot it and unleash their terror upon the bacterium with a ferocity unmatched in the animal world. They swarm against the invader, grabbing it and emptying their granules into the cell until it is killed, as if pumping thousands of shells into the single enemy ship.

But the granulocyte strike force only carries light armament. When they come upon an especially tough invader, one with its own army of millions of bacteria, they empty their ammunition into as many invaders as possible but at the same time know enough to call for reinforcements: the battleships and aircraft carriers of the macrophages.

A *macrophage* is simply a larger, stronger white blood cell. Together with the granulocytes these stronger forces enter the battle and attack relentlessly, to the death. There is no surrender, no negotiation, no standoff. One force wins, and only when its opposition is *totally* destroyed, when not one single cell exists to raise even the weakest resistance. If the invading disease has been reduced from millions of bacteria to a single cell, the armada of granulocytes and macrophages fights on, until that last solitary bacterium has been destroyed. Indeed, even if the enemy wins—as in the case of the person dying of cancer—even if there were only a single macrophage left in the body, it would throw itself into the battle against the overwhelming forces of death, as if it were the last remaining suicide warrior. These white cells are the most loyal and dedicated warriors of all, the Gunga Dins of the immune system.

Complement

The third part of our immune defense is our air force bombers, our armor-piercing shells that actually blow up an invader, as if dropping a bomb into the enemy cell. These are called "complement," a group of nine proteins in our serum that are actually manufactured by the liver (yet another amazingly critical function of this incredible organ). The unique thing with the complement is that it is so fierce in its intent to blow up something that it cannot differentiate between friend and foe. It will bomb anything in sight, healthy cells as well as invading, poisonous ones. Consequently, it needs a "bombsight," a scout to tell it whom to attack and whom to leave alone.

This brings us back to the antibodies. The antibody is like an advance foot soldier who, while shooting at the enemy, is also signaling messages to air support, detailing exactly where to drop their bombs. As the antibody attaches to the marker on the antigen, it also activates the nearest passing unit of complement, which is the first of the nine component proteins. The complement then attaches to the antibody, which in turn signals the second unit of complement to attach to the cell wall. This continues until the ninth unit of complement attaches to the cell wall, at which time the invading cell is blown to smithereens.

To conclude our simplified comparison of the immune system with military action, these three defensive "services"—the army, navy, and air force of our immunity—are, of course, run by the Pentagon. Every action is analyzed and orders are sent to mobilize our various battle forces by the lymph system, the Pentagon of our bodies.

The Lymph System

The *lymph nodes* located throughout our bodies (near our organs, armpits, knees, skin, and practically everywhere) secrete lymphocytes, cells that travel around the body and then return to the lymph nodes. This cycle is continuous. A lymphocyte has no particular locomotive mechanism of its own, yet it lets itself get carried along in the bloodstream, through tissues and organs, muscles and skin, until it eventually gets back to the nearest lymph node, passes through it, and then goes out upon its travels once again. This goes on and on, with some form of the lymphocytes, unlike the granulocytes and macrophages, continuing to live for months and years, making their inspection patrols hundreds of times a day. They apparently do not die, and it is thought by some scientists that they may even live as long as we do. The science of immunology is so young that we still don't understand exactly why a lot of the actions of our immune systems happen. But the lymphocytes make their inevitable rounds day after day, seemingly innocuous, not doing anything but floating through our bodies, bumping along in the traffic of trillions of blood cells.

However, our entire immunology is controlled by these lymphocytes. When a foreign bacterium enters your body, say through a cut on your finger or stepping on a nail at the beach, the antibodies already existing in your system will attack it and prevent infection. Or, if an infection has gained a foothold, the entire system of armed forces will attack and fight it, with the dead bodies forming pus at the site of the battle.

When a new invader appears, one that hasn't been in the body before, it will eventually brush up against one of these circulating lymphocytes. And when it does, that lymphocyte gets excited—so excited that during its brief contact with the invader it makes a "print" or a copy of that antigen's marker and rushes to the nearest lymph node with the information. It is as if a messenger has discovered a spy in the midst of our troops, taken a picture, and rushed to the general to announce the news. The general in the war room, the lymph node, then alerts the entire system. He mobilizes the antibodies and flashes the picture of the marker to them; he alerts the PT-boat navy of granulocytes and their backup battleships, the macrophages, and sends them toward the battle site; he makes sure our bombers, the complement, are getting the proper identification information from the antibodies when they make contact with the antigen. And against especially tough enemies, viruses and parasites that may have strong protective shells around them because they are intracellular microbes (such as the *Progenitor cryptocides* microbe), we even have Green Berets—specially trained "killer" lymphocytes that can attack the invader all by themselves!

As I said, this is an extremely simplified explanation of what is going on within our immune systems, and indeed it can be fun for the sake of instruction to relate it all to a military battle. The main message is that in the final analysis *you* determine whether your forces are well equipped to fight. It is *your* nutrition that manufactures the ammunition necessary for the weapons to work properly. And it was the vaccine that Dr. Virginia administered at her clinic in San Diego that shouted "Cancer! Cancer!" to the generals in the war room.

9

The Discovery of the Cancer Microbe

Warning: this chapter is lengthy and a bit complicated, but Dr. Virginia's slow and tedious process of discovering the cancer microbe is important to understanding further research subsequent to her death. I have tried to simplify the science as best I can.

Progenitor Cryptocides

Dr. Virginia was proud of the fact that she was requested to classify her microorganism in the proper bacteriological fashion at a meeting of the New York Academy of Sciences at the Waldorf-Astoria Hotel in November 1969. Her research team had been describing its discovery of the cancer microorganism, and since all microorganisms are classified into groups according to their unique properties, she was invited to present its proper bacteriological classification. This is called "determinative bacteriology." A classification under a specific name is called "nomenclature." All microorganisms, as most of us learned in high school science, are classified under an order, a family, a genus, a species, and variants.

Thus the microbial agent she believed to be the causative agent in cancer was properly classified at that 1969 meeting as follows:

- Order: Actinomycetales

- Family: Progenitoraceae

- Genus: *Cryptocides*

- Species: *Cryptocides tumefaciens, Cryptocides sclerodermatis* (sclerobacillus), *Cryptocides wilsonii*

- Variants: *Hominii, rodentii, avii,* etc.

What all those impressive words add up to is an increasingly definitive description of the specific microbe. *Actinomycetales,* in Latin, means that the microorganism looks like the sun, having rays or arm-like processes in its growth after being planted on culture media in a laboratory dish, such as the petri dishes many of us used in high school and college biology. Back in school, we learned that "culture media" is simply a biological material that acts as the soil in which the organism grows. (Making the organism grow in such a fashion is called a "culture," or "culturing" the organism.)

Dr. Virginia and her team called the microorganism Progenitoraceae, or "Progenitor," because it appeared to be very primitive in its growth. She explained that forms resembling these organisms have been found in Precambrian rock (between 4.5 billion and 560 million years ago). She also considered it at the source of life, being present in sperm and in developing embryos. Its genus is *Cryptocides,* a combined Greek and Latin word that means "hidden killer." Under "Species" are named the groups, which cause specific diseases, such as cancer, scleroderma (a hardening of the skin), and other connective-tissue diseases. And the "Variants" simply mean that it can occur in several different species, such as man, rodents, birds, and so on. It is important here to remember that she claimed that the Actinomycetales group also contains the microorganisms that cause tuberculosis and leprosy.

Thus, she forever after referred to her cancer microbe as *Progenitor cryptocides,* or *P. cryptocides,* as the proper bacteriological protocol would dictate, or simply as the P.C. microbe. Whichever, the discovery of the microbe as the causative agent in cancer, and the chronology of the development of her theories on how to treat the disease effectively, was, to her and to many others, an exciting, frustrating, and heartbreaking story. She considered herself fortunate enough to have been "in the right place at the right time" quite often. She also had the good fortune during her early days to meet some brilliant researchers and cooperative, pioneering scientists who were not afraid to pursue intuitive pathways that went against the mainstream of popular medical theory. She considered many of these people to have risked their personal reputations and professional standing by continuing to work toward advancing scientific knowledge. As she put it, "There are thousands of so-called terminal cancer patients who are cancer free today, living healthy, vital lives because (the people I associated with) searched for medical truth along the avenues they did, instead of pursuing the safe, well-trod, 'orthodox' boulevards of science."

Important Terms

There are some terms and subtext to be understood before Dr. Virginia's story begins. First, she believed to her dying day that *P. cryptocides* is the ancestral, or primordial, hidden killer implicated in the cause of cancer. Initially, she believed it to be a pathogen only (a disease-producing organism), but with time and further study she realized it was an essential but dormant part of all cells, only activated to repair cell damage. After the repair, it returns to a resting state in the healthy cell, where it remains dormant again. A strong immune system controls this process. However, when immunity is suppressed or weakened, the microbe proliferates and allows cancer to gain a foothold, secreting the same choriogonadotropin hormone found in abundance in all tumors. Hence, as explained more fully later, the microbe is both a "good guy" and a "bad guy," and for this reason is called an "obligate symbiont." (Fear not—I'll never use that term again!)

Another important term is "filterable." In the laboratory, scientists use a Seitz filter (sometimes mistakenly called "Zeitz" or "Zeiss") to initially determine the size of microorganisms. It has been decided that viruses are small enough to pass through the Seitz filter (i.e., are filterable), but that bacteria are too large and cannot pass through. Hence, medical science uses the term "filterable" many times to determine whether an organism is a virus or a bacterium. This is an important term in Dr. Virginia's story because she claimed the cancer-causing microbe she discovered was a bacterium, yet it was small enough to pass through a Seitz filter. This statement is what sends many scientists through the ceiling.

Yet another important term is "acid-fast," or the ability to retain a dye. I'll explain why later, but one of the microbe's significant properties is that of being acid-fast, which means that the microorganism is capable of retaining a certain red dye (called carbolfuchsin), after being washed on a microscope slide with an acid alcohol solution (called decolorization). This trait has allowed researchers to differentiate between this organism and others that are harmless. If an organism is acid-fast, it belongs in the Actinomycetales group and is a first cousin of the lepra and tubercle bacilli.

This method of grouping was discovered accidentally by Robert Koch, M.D., in 1882 when he was studying tuberculosis (TB); it enabled him to identify the tubercle bacillus as its cause. When the acid-fast, red-stained organisms are seen in the sputum of a patient, it means that the patient probably has TB. The same method is applied to nasal smears and tissue preparations from those suspected of having leprosy.

Dr. Koch's subsequent work in inoculating TB patients was at first met with scorn by the established medical community, causing heated medical debate. However, in 1905 he won the Nobel Prize for his tuberculosis work. In 1947, this acid-fast property that enabled Koch to solve the puzzle of TB came quickly to mind when Dr. Virginia found a strange, acid-fast organism present in all the cancers of man and animals that she studied.

Still another important term is "pleomorphic," meaning an organism takes on different physical forms during its life cycle, many of which only vaguely, if at all, resemble any other stage. This phenomenon manifests itself microscopically in the *P. cryptocides* microbe as pinwheels, rods, cotton puffs, donut-shapes, hair-like strands, and several other seemingly unrelated shapes of the same organism.

Until Dr. Virginia claimed to "discover" this allegedly unique organism, the phenomenon of acid-fastness, as it were, was referred to only in the context of Dr. Koch's work with the tubercle bacillus. Though various kinds of cancer organisms had been observed and described by researchers, the universal property of acid-fastness to these organisms was not known. This led Dr. Virginia to consider that she was the first to discover this property; that is, the universal nature of the acid-fast principle, and she immediately began applying this new knowledge to the study of the cause of cancer. She reasoned that if this agent, so obviously related to the TB and leprosy bacilli, was acid-fast, would it cause cancer when injected into laboratory animals? And if so, could the disease itself be treated *with* this bacillus? In other words, could she develop a vaccine from the bacillus; could she *immunize* against cancer using this acid-fast microbe? Further research convinced her that the answer was yes, and from then on her entire future was devoted to proving it.

But the story started much earlier.

Coaxing Clues from Scleroderma

As stated in Chapter 2, Dr. Virginia was graduated from New York University-Bellevue Medical College in 1936, one of only four women doctors in her class. Previously, she had earned three bachelor's degrees in English, History, and Economics from Vassar. However, the influence of her father, Herman W. Wuerthele, M.D., who was one of the early members of the American College of Physicians, and her granduncle, Joseph Benninghof, M.D., a surgeon, had given her a keen interest in medicine.

Soon after graduating from medical school, she met Jack Goldberg, M.D., New York City's Commissioner of Hospitals, and complained that a woman had never been appointed as a resident or a chief intern at a New York hospital. Ten days later, she was called to his office and informed that she was to become New York City's first woman resident physician. While she was elated, the position wasn't *exactly* what she had in mind—she was to be in charge of the prison ward for venereally infected prostitutes! However, she accepted the job, thinking she would at least clear the way for future women residents, and she found it to be one of the most rewarding experiences of her life. Her preconceived notions of the prostitute underwent rapid reevaluation, and she developed great compassion for these women, who were often diseased and discarded by society.

The prison portion of the hospital was located behind a high wall in a compound that also included the infectious disease units of the city hospital. When she attended grand rounds with the other doctors, she had the opportunity to observe several other infectious diseases, especially tuberculosis and leprosy, of which there were many cases in New York City at the time. Even then, when medical science hadn't yet connected them, she sensed that these two infectious diseases were related, and she began reading all the material she could find about them.

Several years later, in 1947, when she was a school physician in Newark, New Jersey, one of the school nurses asked her if she would look at her hands. The nurse had been diagnosed as having Raynaud's syndrome, a disease in which the ends of the fingers become ulcerated. Dr. Virginia noticed that the nurse's fingers appeared pinched and became blue after only mild exposure to cold. There were also areas of hypersensitivity along the nerves of her arms and legs. Upon closer examination Dr. Virginia found a leprosy-like perforation in her septum (the dividing cartilage of the nose). In addition, there were areas of hardness and insensitivity on her skin.

Dr. Virginia's own diagnosis was that she not only had Raynaud's syndrome, but also a condition known as scleroderma. This disorder not only exhibits hardening of the skin but also can involve all of the body's systems and can be fatal in a few years if vital organs are affected.

Enlisting the help of her friends Eva Brodkin, M.D., a dermatologist, and Dr. Camille Mermod, M.D., a pathologist, Dr. Virginia decided to make a full-scale investigation of scleroderma. They made smears from the nurse's nose and finger ulcers and stained them with the acid-fast dyes. To Dr. Virginia's gratified surprise, numerous organisms of the acid-fast type were visible on the slides. She then obtained surgically aseptic specimens of similar affected lesions, stained them, and, deep within the body tissues, just as in leprosy, she again found the same acid-fast microbes.

Dr. Virginia decided that the next step was to make pure cultures of these strange organisms and inject them into chicks and guinea pigs. When she did, most of the animals became diseased— almost all the chicks died, and the guinea pigs developed hard areas of the skin, similar to scleroderma, and some appeared cancerous. Since the incidence of cancer in guinea pigs is only 1 in 500,000, Dr. Virginia considered this observation highly significant.

The Concept

She now reasoned that perhaps scleroderma was a kind of slow cancer. She decided to begin examining cancer tissues with the same method, using the acid-fast Ziehl-Neelsen stain, which is used to identify the tuberculosis organism. In the meantime, she and her team published the original scleroderma papers concerning the sclerobacillus microorganism. (Dr. Virginia claimed this work was later confirmed by Del Motte and Van der Mieren at the Pasteur Institute in Brussels in 1953. In 1971 Alan Cantwell, M.D., a dermatologist at Kaiser-Permanente in Los Angeles, whom I met during my association with Dr. Virginia, independently found the same microorganism and published his work in the *Archives of Dermatology.*)

Dr. Virginia then started collecting all kinds of cancerous tissues directly from operating rooms in her Newark, New Jersey, area. This was to ensure sterility and absolute freshness of the specimens. She soon found that a similar microorganism to the scleroderma bacillus was present in all of them. Growing more excited, she enlisted the assistance of a well-known tissue sectionist in Verona, New Jersey, a Dr. Roy M. Allen, and together they were again able to demonstrate the presence of acid-fast microbes in the cancerous cells. She was delighted that her concept of the parasitization of the cancer cells by these organisms was verified by someone of such repute as Dr. Allen.

Next, Dr. S. J. Rose of St. Michael's Hospital in Newark provided her with a series of unlabeled tissue material. As with the identification of wines in a blindfold wine-tasting today, in every case Dr. Virginia was able to pick out the cancerous tissue from healthy tissue by the presence or absence of the microorganism. Both Dr. Allen and Dr. Rose then joined her in presenting a paper in August 1948 before the New York Microscopical Society, entitled "Microorganisms Associated with Neoplasms."

When Dr. Virginia first conceived of the infectious nature of all cancers, the predominant thought at the time (and even today) was that cancer is caused by a virus. But her *P. cryptocides* bacterium was filterable, which technically classified it as a virus. Sensing criticism on this count, in that early paper she included photomicrographs that further verified the virus-like size of the organism, and showed that the acid-fast microorganisms were present in all forms of human cancer. Since she knew her filterable organism absolutely was a bacterium and not a virus, she knew she was getting into deep water with the medical establishment. (See "News Update: Bacteria Cause Cancer After All," page 121.) In what I found to be typical of Dr. Virginia, she refused to be daunted by what was certain to be a hard, uphill—and personally painful—battle.

The Core Team

It was about this time, in the late 1940s, that Dr. Virginia learned of the work of microbiologist Eleanor Alexander-Jackson, M.D., of Cornell University, who had succeeded in demonstrating that the tubercle bacillus undergoes many changes in morphology (size and shape). She contacted Dr. Alexander-Jackson and the two pioneering women formed an association in which Dr. Alexander-Jackson worked with the tubercle and lepra bacilli, and Dr. Virginia with the *P. cryptocides* bacillus. Dr. Virginia was intrigued with the idea that a bacterium could be so wildly pleomorphic, even existing in a form that didn't resemble a bacterium at all. (Remember, at that time, whether an organism passed through a special filter or not determined whether it was defined as a virus or a bacillus. Viruses, extremely small, passed through; bacilli didn't.) It was then that, whenever Dr. Virginia started referring to her microbe as a bacillus related to the tubercle and lepra bacilli, she was not believed. The professional ridicule had begun.

The newly formed team closed ranks. With Dr. Alexander-Jackson, Dr. Virginia insisted that various experts hear them out. Dr. Alexander-Jackson was working at the laboratory of Wilson Smillie, M.D., at Cornell, and when she and Dr. Virginia explained that they were growing a tumor-producing organism from scleroderma, and that they were convinced there were similar organisms in other collagen diseases, he was about ready to toss Dr. Alexander-Jackson and her strange new colleague out the door. However, one of his physicians saw fit to challenge them. He produced forty anonymous blood samples, some of which had been taken from patients with collagen disease, and some of which were without infection. Dr. Virginia and Dr. Alexander-Jackson soon brought him a 100 percent accurate selection of the twenty-two samples that were infected. This softened up the skeptical Dr. Smillie, and he began to tolerate their work. But he remained skeptical, and apparently kept up the pressure because, according to Dr. Virginia, Dr. Alexander-Jackson soon expressed concern over the future of her work with the tubercle and lepra bacilli in Dr. Smillie's lab. To help save her colleague's job, Dr. Virginia agreed to stop cluttering up the lab and to stay away from Cornell. Instead of the finely equipped university lab, Dr. Virginia then began working in a makeshift laboratory she built in the basement of her home in New Jersey.

The next major event came in 1949: Dr. Virginia's formal affiliation with a major university. She had been working with Abbott Laboratories, using their pharmaceutical and health-care products in developing some of the materials for her further scleroderma work. Since she was achieving some remissions in her patients, Abbott Laboratories agreed to give her a research grant, but with one catch: she'd need a university connection.

Due to state anti-vivisection (animal experimentation) laws at the time, there were no medical schools in New Jersey. However, Rutgers University, in New Brunswick, had numerous branches around the state. Dr. Virginia contacted Royal Schaaf, M.D., president of Newark Presbyterian Hospital, seeking a laboratory in which to conduct her research. Dr. Schaaf offered to give Dr. Virginia the old nurses' residence next door for a laboratory, but only if she could get an affiliation with Rutgers. Armed with this double-barreled backup, she saw her chance for the grant and met with James Allison, Ph.D., director of the Bureau of Biological Research at Rutgers. He had corresponded with her in the past, expressing interest in her work and complimenting her on the confirmation she had received from various associates. He was therefore most knowledgeable about her experimental goals and cooperative. On June 2, 1949, she was named head of the new Rutgers Presbyterian Hospital Laboratory for the Study of Proliferative Diseases, Bureau of Biological Research, Rutgers University. Her Abbott Laboratories grant was on its way.

The nurses' residence wasn't much to work with. It resembled an old Victorian brownstone, was in terrible repair, and needed serious renovation. It was Rutgers' feeling that if Dr. Virginia and her team rehabilitated the building and started up some serious research work, they would be able to attract still more grants besides the Abbott Laboratories funds. Dr. Virginia once again killed the proverbial pair of birds with the single stone. She not only raised funds through the gracious help of a local, extremely zealous woman, but the woman, in turn, induced the local labor unions to volunteer time and material to turn the nurses' residence into a clean, efficient laboratory.

As a result of the refurbishment, Dr. Virginia and Rutgers applied for a number of substantial grants; these financed her work for the next three years. She received grants from the American Cancer Society, the Damon Runyon Fund, the Rosenwald Foundation, *Reader's Digest*, Charles Pfizer & Company, Lederle Laboratories, a second grant from Abbott Laboratories, and many private individuals.

The next few years at Rutgers were to be the most significant period of her work in cancer research. She and her colleagues were enthusiastic that their work would prove once and for all that the *P. cryptocides* microbe was the cause of cancer and that a vaccine could be made to defend against it.

Proof of the Cancer-Causing Microbe

Now that Dr. Virginia had the necessary facilities at Newark, under Rutgers University auspices, she was able to expand her operation as each of the abovementioned grants came in. She was named an associate professor in the Bureau of Biological Research and proceeded to build her research team. Dr. Eleanor Alexander-Jackson was her first choice.

While Dr. Virginia was trying to set herself up with a lab in New Jersey, Dr. Alexander-Jackson had decided to research cancer infection for herself and had obtained fresh tumors under sterile conditions from Memorial Hospital at Cornell. After studying the cultures from these tumors she confirmed that the specific organism, *P. cryptocides*, was present in all the tumors she examined. It wasn't hard after that for Dr. Virginia to convince her friend to leave Cornell and join her at Rutgers. Dr. Alexander-Jackson commuted daily from New York to work in the lab as Dr. Virginia's bacteriologist. The rest of the team consisted of Dr. Roy Allen, the histologist, who kept himself, and an assistant busy preparing tissue sections of material; Dr. Lawrence W. Smith, a pathologist; Joseph Patti, an experienced animal-tumor expert from a distinguished institute in New York (Dr. Virginia couldn't remember the name); Marilyn Clark, a tissue culturist; and Andrew Steciuw, who cared for the experimental animals.

In the five years from 1949 to 1953 a great deal was accomplished. Dr. Virginia was assigned a number of hospital beds to which she could bring cancer patients for study, and she had access to fresh cancer material from the hospital operating rooms. She had the full cooperation of the Presbyterian Hospital under Dr. Schaaf, and of Rutgers University itself, under Dr. Allison. She collected and studied all the obtainable animal tumors believed to be infectious in nature and supposedly caused by a virus. They were the Rous, Walker, Sprague-Dawley, Shope, and sarcoma-180 tumors, plus various types of fowl neoplasia. From these she made cultures, bacterial isolates, that she compared with cultures derived from many types of fresh, uncontaminated human tumors from the blood and other body fluids of patients with advanced cancer.

As anticipated, these cultures had a great similarity to one another. There were some variations as to size and some differences in the kind of media or material in which they would grow. Certain strains fermented one kind of sugar; some others. Some could live with little or no oxygen; some required more. Dr. Alexander-Jackson studied various peptones, or protein fractions, until she found those that were best for producing good growth of the organisms in test tubes. Dr. Virginia worked with making a medium from chick embryos.

According to Dr. Virginia, all of these culture studies strongly supported the growth of the organism. Over and over, her *P. cryp-*

tocides organisms were acid-fast and highly pleomorphic in their growth pattern. They stained with the Ziehl-Neelsen stain in the same way as did the tubercle bacillus. The bacteriologists at Rutgers University were satisfied that she had pure cultures free of contamination from other bacteria. (Contamination is always the most important problem in the isolation of microorganisms. Contaminants are present everywhere. Usually, they are harmless bacteria from the air or soil, or from humans or animals. The danger is that they may simulate the real culprits, the pathogens, that is, the disease producers. No laboratory is ever free of them. In fact, it was the contamination of Sir Alexander Fleming's cultures by the penicillin mold that led to his famous discovery of penicillin.)

For that reason, Dr. Virginia's cultures were scrutinized repeatedly. Strains of the *P. cryptocides* were sent to many laboratories for identification, but none could really classify them, because at the time they were totally unknown. They had many forms, but they always evolved into the same microbe no matter how often they were cultured. The microbes resembled the mycobacteria more than anything else. (The tubercle bacillus is a mycobacterium or fungoid bacillus.) When her advisers at Rutgers felt that she had pure, uncontaminated cultures, her team was ready to test them against Koch's law, or postulates.

This was a critically important facet of Dr. Virginia's hypothesis, because Koch's law is the accepted foolproof method of proving the cause of a disease. Koch's postulates are:

1. The microorganism must be present in every case of the disease.

2 It must be possible to cultivate the microorganism outside the host (i.e., animal) in some artificial medium.

3. The inoculation of this culture must produce the disease in a susceptible animal.

4. The microorganism must then be re-obtained from these inoculated animals and cultured again.

Dr. Virginia was able to fulfill Koch's postulates, which was a truly exciting development. Dr. Virginia and her team realized its significance because if she claimed that her microbe caused cancer and the microbe fulfilled Koch's postulates, then the medical community surely should sit up and take notice.

The culmination of this work was published by Dr. Virginia and Dr. Alexander-Jackson, plus four other authors, in the *American Journal of Medical Sciences* in December 1950, more than half a century ago. It was entitled "Cultural Properties and Pathogenicity of Certain Microorganisms Obtained from Various Proliferative and Neoplastic Diseases." The other authors sported impressive credentials indeed: Dr. John A. Anderson, head of the Department of Bacteriology at Rutgers; Dr. James Hillier, developer of the electron microscope and head of electron microscopy at RCA Victor Laboratories in Princeton, New Jersey; Dr. Roy M. Allen, noted histologist; and Dr. Lawrence W. Smith, noted pathologist and author of a well-known pathology textbook then used in medical colleges.

This paper was the final result of several years of effort, starting with Dr. Virginia's early scleroderma work in the mid-1940s. It underwent three months of scrutiny by the Rutgers group headed by Drs. Allison and Anderson before passing their rigid requirements for publication. At the time of my association with Dr. Virginia to gather material for her book, I checked with a few scientists of my acquaintance, who, in turn, researched the paper, and they corroborated its significance. It is my understanding that it still stands as a milestone treatise on the infectious nature of cancer.

The paper described how pure cultures were obtained from the various cancers of both human beings and animals. These were then injected into animals capable of being infected. Gradually, diseased areas developed that resembled those from which the cultures were obtained. Then pure cultures were re-isolated from the infected animals. Koch's postulates were fulfilled to the satisfaction of Dr. Virginia and the entire team, and to that of her biology superiors at Rutgers.

NEWS UPDATE:
BACTERIA CAUSE CANCER AFTER ALL

Dr. Virginia was roundly derided for suggesting that her microorganism *P. cryptocides* not only was the causative agent for cancer, but also that it was a bacterium, not a virus. However, back in 2002, Dr. Juanita Merchant, a University of Michigan gastroenterologist, published a report that implicated *Helicobacter pylori,* a bacterium, in the development of stomach cancer. Since then, research in many reputable institutions has shown that *H. pylori* is in fact a precursor not only to stomach cancer, but also to pancreatic cancer, lymphoma, esophageal cancer, and colon cancer.

In a 2013 study published in *Gut Microbes,* Dr. Dana Hardbower and associates at the Vanderbilt University Medical Center referred to the *H. pylori* bacterium as the "smoking gun" for gastric cancer. The first sentence of their abstract states, "*Helicobacter pylori* is the leading risk factor associated with gastric carcinogenesis."

Normally, the strong acids in the stomach kill off the various viruses, bacteria, and other microorganisms present. However, researchers discovered that *H. pylori* actually thrive in the savage stomach environment. In recent years there have been lots of studies demonstrating the *H. pylori*–gastric cancer link. In 1994, the International Agency for Research on Cancer created a controversy by classifying *H. pylori* as a carcinogen, but since then, colonization of the stomach with *H. pylori* has been increasingly accepted as an important risk factor for gastric cancers. Now, according to the National Cancer Institute (NCI), infection with *H. pylori* is the most important risk factor for gastric cancer and lymphoma.

Moreover, also according to the NCI, it has been observed that many people who had surgery to treat peptic ulcers developed pancreatic cancer up to twenty years later. In addition, one study found that out of 92 pancreatic cancer patients, 65 percent tested positive for *H. pylori,* while only 45 percent of non-cancer control participants tested positive. The study, published in the NCI's journal in 2001, concluded, "A positive association exists between *H. pylori* and pancreatic cancer."

There is much more evidence surfacing that bacteria may be involved in carcinogenesis. Since completion of the Human Genome Project in 2003, an international research effort to study the genetics of disease, there have been many studies of viral DNA and its implication in the initiation of cancer formation, but the question of bacterial DNA had been ignored. Researchers from the University of Maryland reported evidence in *National Science Foundation News* (June 20, 2013) that bacterial DNA inserted into human chromosomes may play a role in carcinogenesis.

In the June 2013 issue of *Nature,* Dr. Shin Yoshimoto of the Japanese Center for Cancer Research in Tokyo studied microbes in the microbiome (the 100 trillion bacteria that live in the gut), and concluded in his experiments that there is a causative relationship between certain gut bacteria in obese mice and liver cancer.

Also, in 2013, the journal *Cancer Research* reported that researchers at the University of California, Los Angeles, Jonsson Comprehensive Cancer Center, discovered that certain types of bacteria present in the intestinal tract are major contributors to lymphomas.

Finally, two studies at the Harvard School of Public Health in Boston and at Case Western Reserve University School of Dental Medicine in Cleveland have shown how bacteria that are sometimes found in the mouth and gut can fuel the development of bowel cancer. The studies show how stomach bacteria called fusobacteria (*Fusobacterium nucleatum*) can stimulate immune responses and turn on cancer growth genes. Both research results were published in 2013 in the journal *Cell Host and Microbe.*

Again, bacteria? Causing cancer? Dr. Virginia isn't rolling in her grave—she's dancing!

Cancer as a Systemic Disease

The next step was to prove that the cancerous growth itself was not the whole disease. Dr. Virginia explained to me that for more than 100 years, people like Rudolf Virchow, M.D., known as the father of modern pathology, thought that cancer cells themselves were parasites within the body. He did not understand that the small coccus-like granules he saw dividing in the cancers were not the development of daughter cells within mother cells, but that instead they represented the true intracellular parasite that was the causative agent. In his book *The Savage Cell*, author Patrick McGrady defines cancer as "a savage cell which somehow evades the laws of the body, corrupts the forces which normally protect the body, invades the well-ordered society of cells that surrounds it, colonizes distant areas, and as a finale to its cannibalistic orgy of flesh consuming flesh, commits suicide by destroying its host." This is a picturesque and dramatic description of the cancer cell, but Dr. Virginia considered it not entirely true. The whole truth, she conjectured, may be that the parasite within the cancer transforms the normal cell into a sick cell that cannot mature by normal cell growth processes. In other words, the tumor itself is not the disease.

Dr. Virginia pointed out by way of analogy that no one today believes that the pleomorphic lesions of syphilis, which can appear anywhere in or on the body of an untreated person, constitute the disease itself. Volumes have been written about the cause and cure of syphilis. The effects of the disease, like cancer, have reached into every corner of the civilized world. Mighty kings fathered syphilitic weaklings. The stigma of syphilis that bridged generations was even the basis for Henrik Ibsen's famous play *Ghosts*.

Then in 1905, zoologist Fritz Schaudinn, M.D., found the cause, the spirochete *Treponema pallidum*. The microbe causes the disease! The search for the cure began: injections of arsenicals, mercury, and bismuth, to name but a few. These were often dangerous and not always effective. Such treatments gave rise to the famous saying, "One night with Venus and ten years with Mercury." Then in 1928 came Sir Alexander Fleming's great discovery. We can now say "Syphilis? Penicillin!" All is said in two words.

Bacteriologist Francisco Duran-Reynals, M.D., in the years from 1940 to 1956, showed that the Rous "virus," or tumor agent, could cause acute and lethal hemorrhagic disease when given in large amounts, but smaller amounts could lead to a lesser reaction result-ing in cancer. With a still further repression of the tumor infectious agent, chronic, interstitial disease similar to arthritis and heart dis-ease would appear in his experimental animals. Dr. Duran-Reynals also proved that the Rous "virus" can cross species barriers and infect ducks and turkeys, and that filtrates—that is, filtered mate-rial from tumor tissue, not the cells themselves—can transmit Rous sarcoma to guinea pigs, rabbits, and marmosets.

Dr. Virginia's paper, "Cultural Properties and Pathogenicity of Certain Microorganisms Obtained from Various Proliferative and Neoplastic Diseases," proved that the tumor was not the disease. She claimed her paper bore out her insistence that it was the *P. cryp-tocides* that caused the disease in the animals and so fulfilled Koch's postulates. Hence, it does appear that in 1948 she was years ahead of others in showing that the Rous tumor agent was not a virus but a pleomorphic bacterium. And she claimed Dr. Rous's "tumor agent" was the *P. cryptocides* microbe. As in Duran-Reynals's work, the tumors were only a part of the resultant disease.

In addition to tumors, there were cheesy lesions or areas resem-bling tuberculosis, which could invade any one of the essential organs such as the liver, kidney, heart, or lung. These organs might show changes in the connective tissue, called collagen, that could lead to degeneration as seen in the chronic human degenerative dis-eases. It was Dr. Virginia's further conclusion that these microor-ganisms, *P. cryptocides*, could not only cause cancer but also a number of other ailments that afflict people. The infectious nature of arthritis, of some kinds of heart, liver, and kidney impairment, and most recently diabetes, has been proposed. Dr. Virginia always alleged that many medical researchers would admit that the patterns of these diseases point to their latent infectious nature, but that no one had come forth with an antigen or actual causative agent. Because she claimed that it was these filterable forms of the *P. cryptocides* microbe that have been described as C-particles, mycoplasma, or viruses by other research workers, she proposed that certain strains of the *Progenitor* group were, in fact, the culprits.

Before the theory that the filterable form of the *Progenitor* group was equivalent to the so-called tumor-viruses could be proven, it was necessary for Dr. Virginia to spend many months working with the aforementioned Dr. Hillier of the RCA Victor Laboratories in Princeton, New Jersey. There the bacterial cultures isolated from human and animal tumors were passed through filters that permitted passage only of so-called true viruses. These filtrates contained minute forms of life, which then re-grew to become bacterial cultures. This work proved conclusively that the Rous agent was not a virus. Peyton Rous, M.D., did not call his tumor filtrates "viruses," but "filterable microbial agents," or "tumor agents." A true virus has been defined as a submicroscopic infectious unit that lives only in the presence of living cells and cannot exist even momentarily outside them. But the Rous "tumor agents" could be dried, stored on a shelf at room temperature for years, and when mixed with saline could then be reactivated to initiate fresh tumors.

Therefore, these "tumor agents" were definitely *not* viruses, she concluded. A great deal of time and effort had been spent in trying to find a virus implicated in any form of human cancer. *None had yet been proven.* However, Dr. Virginia was proposing that the filterable forms of *P. cryptocides*, which are of virus size, are the causative agents in human and animal cancers, and that, like the Rous tumor agents, they are transmissible from one animal to another. There was some criticism in those days stating that mice often developed cancer spontaneously and that therefore it would be better to work with other animals as well. However, in all research the results are judged by the comparison of the treated animal with the untreated controls, so that even if there are cancers in the untreated, there is a significant differential. The need for genetically controlled mice led to the development of certain inbred strains having predictable sites and numbers of tumors. Dr. Virginia also used these strains as well as guinea pigs, which have a natural immunity and are resistant to cancer. Because, as stated previously, only 1 guinea pig in 500,000 develops cancer spontaneously, it was significant that Dr. Virginia was able to produce tumors in an amazing 25 percent.

It was while working with guinea pigs that her suspicions as to the method of transmissibility of tumors were confirmed. Due to an error, the infected guinea pigs were housed in cages at the top of the laboratory animal racks, while the healthy, uninoculated controls, instead of being housed on different racks, were placed in cages underneath. To Dr. Virginia's surprise, the control animals also developed cancer. On careful inspection she found that droppings from the top cages sometimes fell into the drinking water and food of the guinea pigs below. From that time on, she kept the controls in separate rooms. She further observed that when her animal caretaker changed his gown, cap, mask, and gloves before going from one area to the other, the guinea pig controls thereafter stopped developing cancer.

The observation was dramatic indeed, and her convictions about the transmissibility of cancer continued to grow.

Dr. Virginia continued to ascertain the effect of her cancer cultures on living tissue cultures, that is, on uncontaminated, totally clean tissue in test tubes (in vitro). These tissues were living cells nourished by various types of nutritive material, some artificial and some taken from serum of chickens and calves. She found that under the influence of the microbes the tissue cultures showed marked changes, such as degeneration and destruction of cells with abnormal cell division. However, she suspected that since the embryo fluids used for nourishing the tissue cultures came from chicks, they might contain the cancer agent. This proved to be the case, since many chickens and their eggs have the pathogenic form of the cancer microbe.

Thereafter, whenever "spontaneous" conversion of a tissue culture to the cancerous state was described in the literature, she would be most skeptical as to the cause. Again, it was the difference between the infected and the uninfected tissue cultures that was significant in short-term studies. (Later, Dr. Irene Corey Diller of the Department of Pathology at the Institute for Cancer Research, and Dr. William F. Diller, of the Department of Biology, University of Pennsylvania, were to perform some excellent experiments with cancer cultures in living tissue, which confirmed the conversion of normal cells to abnormal cells by the inoculation of the *P. cryptocides* cancer microbes into the tissue culture of cells.)

Dr. Virginia once told me that at times the work that she and Dr. Alexander-Jackson did was sad and unpleasant. At one point it occurred to her that it was important to study one kind of human cancer thoroughly. She and Dr. Alexander-Jackson decided that the cancer of the human breast would be the most suitable, since such cancers usually were enclosed within the breast and not subject to contamination from the bowel or adjacent structures. Also, they were a common type of cancer and not too difficult to obtain. It became Dr. Virginia's sad job to collect thirty breasts that had been removed for cancer from the operating rooms. They were fresh from the surgeon's knife, obtained directly after the pathologist had taken specimens for sectioning. They were, of course, kept sterile. She brought them back to the laboratory, where she and Dr. Alexander-Jackson dissected the cancers and the glands from under the armpit, called the axilla. They numbered the specimens, cultured not only the tumors but the glands as well, and compared them with the pathologists' reports. In *all* of the cases where they could obtain blood samples, they grew positive cultures from the blood. Also, even when the pathologist reported that the underarm glands were negative for tumor cells, the cancer organisms developed from them when cultured. The two scientists concluded that *the results showed that cancer is not a localized, but a generalized (systemic) disease.*

A Cure in a Potential Vaccine

Later, in March 1953, when Dr. Virginia's group was invited to present papers at the Sixth International Congress of Microbiology in Rome, she invited an exceptionally well-trained pathologist from Scranton, Pennsylvania, George Clark, M.D., to attend with her. Thirty-three years before, in 1920, Dr. Clark had reported on the successful culturing of a Glover's cancer organism and the development of metastasizing tumors in animals brought on by injections of human malignancy cultures. Dr. Virginia was certain that what he had called the "Glover organism" in 1920 was undoubtedly the same as her organism.

However, most of the work of Dr. Thomas Glover, a Canadian, was unpublished. When Dr. Clark and his associates were invited to Washington, D.C., to repeat the experiments, under the supervision of George W. McCoy, M.D., Director of Public Health, they remained there for eight years and their work, too, was never published. Dr. Virginia was perplexed as to why, but we never followed it up.

At the Rome congress, Dr. Clark presented a scholarly paper. It was gratifying to Dr. Virginia that after many sacrifices, tribulations, and the suppression of his work, she could give Dr. Clark the opportunity to present it to a distinguished audience. Prior to the Rome meeting, they all met in Scranton to compare notes with earlier workers, such as Drs. Jacob Engle, H. B. Leffler, and M. J. Scott. The team also raised sufficient funds to bring Dr. Franz Gerlach from Germany to be honored in Scranton at a "Gerlach Day" celebration. He had devoted much of his life in Vienna to the study of the cancer parasite, which he called a "micromycete." (Dr. Virginia never missed a chance to espouse her conviction that there was no place in research for jealousy or destructive competition. She often railed about how often a truth has been suppressed or recognition delayed because selfish peers would not recognize the merit of a fellow worker!)

While Dr. Clark was visiting, he reported to Dr. Virginia that Dr. Glover had been able to produce antibodies and antiserum in sheep and horses that were beneficial in the treatment of human cancer. Using Glover's method, the team decided to try to reproduce his work by immunizing sheep with an attenuated, or weakened, culture. Harriette Vera, Ph.D., chief bacteriologist at, and one of the owners of, the Baltimore Biological Laboratories, who had done much of the confirmatory work with Dr. Virginia's cultures, sent her a generous contribution that enabled her to perform this experiment.

As Dr. Virginia described it, first she needed an area in which to keep her experimental animals. She had a patient in Nutley, New Jersey, who owned a dairy farm, and who agreed to rent her a small remote pasture. Then she purchased a flock of twenty sheep and engaged a state veterinarian to assist her. He examined the sheep and found them free of disease. She attenuated some of the stock vaccines she had on hand, such as cultures from human breast cancer, from the sarcoma of a young boy, from a human leukemia, from the Rous chicken tumor, from arthritis, and from fowl leukosis. She then injected two sheep with each strain. After about four weeks, the veterinarian reported that some of the sheep were getting sick. They examined the sheep weekly and provided the veterinarian with the attenuated vaccines from the cancer cultures, which he used for immunization. Several ewes aborted their young. The fetuses were macerated. Some of the sheep developed very swollen painful joints and could scarcely graze. Others looked sickly and got thin. Dr. Virginia and her colleagues realized that the organisms in their vaccines were still alive, and not dead as they should have been to make a weak enough vaccine for immunization without actually giving the sheep a disease. In other words, they had not fully immunized the sheep, but had given them the disease with the living organisms in their vaccine. They then asked the veterinarian to bleed the sheep in order to assay their serum for antibodies. They received the sterile sera, but the sheep had to be destroyed and carried away for incineration. Dr. Virginia was so concerned that the soil of the farmer's pasture might be contaminated that she persuaded the Nutley Fire Department to burn over the entire field, including all the fodder that had been given to the sheep. Nature would have to do the rest in sterilizing the soil.

Although the sheep had to be destroyed, Dr. Virginia thought she learned a great deal from that seemingly failed experiment. For example, she said she learned that the chicken vaccine agglutinated (formed into glue-like clumps) in high dilution with the cultures from the boy's sarcoma. Also, she learned that breast cancer serum reacted with the human leukemia isolates. And she learned that the Rous sarcoma serum reacted with all of the cultures. This meant that the human cultures cross-reacted with one another strongly and also cross-reacted with the animal serum samples, showing that tumors are not specific to certain organs or species. In other words, *the tumors could be transmitted from one type of tissue to another, from one kind of animal to another.*

She next turned her attention to fowl leukosis, a cancerous disease that was killing many fowl on the poultry farms of New Jersey. She took her team to Verona, New Jersey, to interview a chicken rancher she knew, because he had told her that he was losing about 25 percent of his chickens to fowl leukosis. She asked him if she might have some of his sick birds, and he handed her three chickens that could no longer stand up. She took them to the laboratory, and in a short time they were dead. She then took samples of their hearts' blood, which grew into the same kind of cultures as those derived from all her other tumors.

Dr. Virginia decided that this time she would completely inactivate the cultures. Meaning, she would be sure that the microbes were killed before she used them to produce antibodies, this time in rabbits. She thoroughly immunized two sets of rabbits; one set with a tissue vaccine made from the tumor, and the other one with a bacterial vaccine made from the cultured microbes, both from the chickens. She bled the rabbits and refrigerated the serum. Then she went back to the Verona rancher and asked him for six more dying chickens. All six were so weak they could no longer stand. Their heads fell over, and they lay on their sides twitching from time to time, their beaks open.

She separated the chickens into three groups of two. The two she didn't treat died before morning. Another two were treated with the rabbit antiserum produced by tumor cell vaccine, and the last pair were treated with the rabbit antiserum from the bacterial vaccine. The team then watched the chickens carefully. Dr. Virginia said that in just a few hours all four got up on their legs and were able to drink water. She treated them for several days with all the rabbit serum she had. All four recovered completely. The ones that received the tissue vaccine recovered more slowly and were somewhat stunted in growth. The two chickens treated with the bacterial vaccine became very vigorous, full-fleshed roosters. After several months she destroyed the stunted birds. But the team was ecstatic—the birds were tumor-free! The other two roosters were kept for one year, and they reportedly remained perfectly clear of any tumors.

Dr. Virginia then told me about making rounds one day in the hospital, when one of the patients remarked, "You'd think we were out in the country instead of in the middle of the city. Every morning at daylight a couple of roosters crow so loudly we're all awakened out of a sound sleep. I wonder who's keeping them in the neighborhood?"

She took the hint. When one of the janitors remarked that they were mighty fine looking birds and would make a nice dinner for someone, Dr. Virginia gave them to him for his Christmas dinner. She knew that he could never find such beautiful birds anywhere on the market. She thought that whatever fowl he might have bought for dinner would have been infected with cancer, but her rabbit antiserum had cured the cancer in her chickens.

Most important, Dr. Virginia concluded proudly, it was the anti-serum produced in the rabbits with the pure bacterial *P. cryplocides* culture that was the curative agent.

10

Building the Team

Although the research work Dr. Virginia was doing was being confirmed by many corroborative workers, she contended that there continued to be considerable friction between her group and the groups that directed their efforts toward the cancer cell itself instead of toward the microbic cause of cancer. Their theory was that if you could destroy the cancer cell, you could conquer the disease. This was essentially the theory that Rudolf Virchow had proposed so many years ago when he posited that the cancer cell acts parasitically upon the body, and one has only to destroy it to cure the cancer. This is a completely erroneous principle that still persists today.

How many patients over the years have asked in complete bewilderment, "Doctor, why has my cancer come back? They said they got it all, and now it is spread all over."

Dr. Virginia's answer, invariably, was, "Immunity!"

Dr. Virginia contended that the complete removal of the tumor, as explained in Chapter 7, may have some influence upon the course of the disease, but it is not the determining factor in the survival of the patient. "Immunity is the answer!" was her invariable retort. If a patient's immune system is not at maximum strength, she insisted, the smallest tumor completely removed will not prevent other tumors from arising in other parts of the body.

The Politics of Cancer

At the time of her Rutgers discoveries, many of the large research centers, such as the Memorial Sloan-Kettering Cancer Center in New York City, were dedicated largely to finding a chemical or group of chemicals that would destroy the cancer *cell*. Her opinion at the time was that Cornelius P. Rhoads, M.D., then director of Memorial Sloan-Kettering, would brook no competition or interference from anyone who disagreed with his concepts along this line. He considered her and her collaborators as an upstart group. He was often heard to say, "When the cause and cure of cancer is found, I will find it." Dr. Virginia thought he died a disappointed man.

It is always amazing how the fallacious conclusions of researchers associated with large, heavily endowed institutions can sway the minds of scientists and physicians all over the world. Dr. Virginia thought this was the case with Dr. Rhoads. The Memorial Sloan-Kettering Cancer Center was heavily endowed with millions of dollars from private industrial giants, and she thought Rhoads wielded his authority like a heavy club. She claimed that he himself was less a scientist than a promoter and a politician determined to perpetuate the powerful cancer interests vested in him and his institution.

According to Dr. Virginia, Dr. Rhoads was committed to chemotherapy, since he was head of chemical warfare during most of World War II. She thought he tried to turn the war's chemical warfare against the cancer cell within the human body. She said his great mistake was that he believed the cancer cell to be the causative agent of the disease, and not the parasite contained *within* the cell. To her, "unleashing the horrors of chemical warfare and the atomic bomb" in the form of chemotherapy and cobalt radiation against the helpless victims of a microbic disease was illogical. Further, she considered Dr. Rhoads not content to limit his theories to his own institution, but determined to dictate the research policies of the entire country. At one point, Dr. Virginia contended, he almost succeeded in destroying the basic biological research at the Institute for Cancer Research in Philadelphia and turning the institute into a subservient satellite. Fortunately, she said, he failed.

About 1950, Irene Diller, Ph.D., of that same Institute for Cancer Research in Philadelphia attempted to set up a symposium at the New York Academy of Sciences in order to present a number of papers concerning her work on the microbic infectious nature of cancer. The meeting was killed by Dr. Rhoads.

In Dr. Virginia's words, "All he needed was something to discredit one of us. Dr. Diller had accepted from a commercial company several ultraviolet sterilizing lights for her laboratory. There were no strings attached. However, Dr. Rhoads used her acceptance of this gift to state that she had 'commercialized' her work and therefore was not eligible to sponsor a symposium." (It was to be almost twenty years later, 1969, before she finally held her symposium at the New York Academy of Sciences.)

Standing by What They Believed

At her house one evening, Dr. Virginia told me the following story:

> One day in 1951, Eleanor [Dr. Alexander-Jackson] said to me, "I hate to bring this up, Virginia, but I have a lump in my left breast." She came over to my office, where I examined her. She certainly did have a sizable hard mass in the inner upper quadrant of her left breast. There was no question in my mind as to what it was. Frank Adair, M.D., at Sloan-Kettering arranged for her to have surgery. The tumor was malignant, and Eleanor underwent a radical mastectomy. Her father, Dr. Jerome Alexander, and I stood by anxiously during the surgery. While we were waiting, I was summoned over the loudspeaker to Dr. Rhoads's office. I went there immediately. Dr. Rhoads motioned me to a chair in his large, luxurious office overlooking East Sixty-eighth Street. He was an imposing man, tall and quite handsome.

"You people can help us a great deal with our research," he said. I thought to myself, how ironic—now that Eleanor herself is afflicted with the disease, he has softened and will be more cooperative in our work. Then he continued, "We've been looking for a tumor such as she has—one on the inner side of the breast where the glands drain and the tumor lying within the mediastinum. (This is an area between the lungs where the great vessels come from the heart. It is fairly inaccessible.)

"We would like to have someone try out a new surgical technique," he continued. "She could be the first one to have her sternum (the breast bone) split, permitting us to do a dissection around the heart and great vessels to remove the glands there. We have not been able to get permission from anyone for this surgery. She would be performing a great service in permitting us to do this, as it would be an experiment to see how it would affect a patient and to determine the length of time she might survive."

I was speechless. Dr. Rhoads wanted me to talk Eleanor into having the experimental operation! This man had been discrediting my research at every turn, and now he was talking about my dear friend and loyal colleague as if she were a laboratory animal. I was infuriated.

"Not on your life!" I told him. "That is a cruel and disfiguring operation. Her body could be so shocked that she might not even withstand the operation. She doesn't even *need* a radical, since her glands don't drain toward the axilla. I will oppose the idea with every ounce of persuasion I have."

I left the room with tears in my eyes. Dr. Rhoads had not called me to his office to commiserate, to sympathize, or to help, but only to ask that my friend Eleanor be sacrificed on his political altar of research.

Eleanor came through the surgery splendidly. The next day when I told her what Dr. Rhoads wanted me to suggest to her, she was most indignant. "We should stand by what we believe," she said sternly. "I won't have any cobalt treatments or any further surgery. I'll watch my diet and take our vaccines." This she did. It is now more than thirty years since that fateful day. Eleanor tells me she has never had the slightest evidence of a return of her tumor. She recuperated rapidly and was back at the laboratory in a short time. Eleanor has always been a woman of great stamina and determination. Her daily trips to the Newark laboratory in the freezing cold or the blazing heat were feats of endurance. It took at least one and a half hours from her apartment on Riverside Drive to the laboratory. She was always cheerful, eager, and interested in our work. Every step of the way was a great adventure that we shared. Sometimes we differed and quarreled; sometimes one felt put upon by the other, but reason always shone through. Our friendship has continued all these years. Though we are very different people, we have been held together by our interest in the microbial nature of cancer, and each by faith in the integrity and good judgment of the other. My admiration for her father, Dr. Jerome Alexander, was profound. He was not only a brilliant chemist but also a great humanitarian.

When Dr. Virginia told me that story, in the quiet of her capacious La Jolla living room, there were tears in her eyes. While she was always passionately involved in her patients' welfare, it was the only time in our association that I saw her so overcome with emotion. There were also tears in the eyes of her devoted husband, Dr. Owen Wheeler.

A Network of Support

During the Rutgers years Dr. Virginia and her team made every effort to coordinate their work with related microbial procedures. They visited a number of scientists who were interested in their approach to the cancer problem. In 1949, before Rutgers would consider accepting her projects under their auspices, Dr. James Allison and she had traveled to Philadelphia to meet Dr. Margaret Lewis, M.D., at the Wistar Institute. Dr. Lewis and her husband had spent a lifetime of research in the microbiology of cancer. A great deal of their work had been done with the rat, and Dr. Lewis had stored paraffin blocks of experimental rat cancer in her laboratory. After they had conversed for some time, Dr. Virginia said, "You can give me any one of those tumor blocks, and I will demonstrate with proper staining the causative organisms in the sections."

Dr. Lewis gave her a block of tissue from the shelf at random. Even without the corroboration of the stained slides, she told Dr. Allison that she thought Dr. Virginia's work should be associated with Rutgers University. Dr. Virginia in turn gave the tissue block over to Dr. Roy Allen, who prepared the sections with her special stains. As expected, the hidden killer *P. cryptocides* was revealed throughout the tumor by the acid-fast stain. The stained sections were then sent to Dr. Lewis and Dr. Allison for their own use.

After Dr. Eleanor Alexander-Jackson joined the laboratory, they continued to visit various clinics and research centers. Dr. Virginia was especially interested in meeting with Elise L'Esperance, M.D., of what was then the Strang Memorial Cancer Detection Clinic in New York City. Not only had she founded the world's first cancer detection clinic, but she also had worked on the microbic theory of cancer. Dr. Virginia recalled that when she was a student at Bellevue Medical College, a pathology professor had said rather disparagingly, "There is a woman pathologist at Cornell who thinks Hodgkin's disease (a form of glandular cancer) is caused by avian tuberculosis. She has published a report on this, but no one has confirmed her findings."

As Dr. Virginia looked into the microscope at the slides of Hodgkin's disease, she couldn't help comparing them with the slides she had seen of tuberculosis. In Hodgkin's disease, the large multinucleated giant cells are called Reed-Sternberg cells. They are similar to the giant cells of tuberculosis. In tuberculosis these cells form and engulf the tubercle bacilli. Dr. Virginia entertained the thought that Dr. L'Esperance was probably right, but also that she would have a difficult time gaining acceptance. Years later, after she had made her initial observations of the acid-fast tuberculosis-like forms in scleroderma, followed by observations of the same forms in all cancers including Hodgkin's disease, Dr. Virginia remembered Dr. L'Esperance's theory about Hodgkin's disease and avian tuberculosis.

Sometime in 1950, while she was at the Newark laboratory, Dr. Virginia telephoned Dr. L'Esperance. The latter said she would be glad to see her and Dr. Alexander-Jackson. They agreed to meet at the Strang Memorial Cancer Detection Clinic (now the Strang Cancer Prevention Center). Dr. Virginia knew something about the founding of the Strang Center and was most anxious to see the clinic. Dr. L'Esperance had been very active for years at the New York Women's Infirmary, where she established her first cancer detection center. She and her sister, May Strang, were nieces and heirs of Chauncey Depew, president of the New York Central Railroad and a famous after-dinner speaker. After his death the two women inherited a great deal of money. They founded the Kate Depew Strang Memorial Cancer Detection Clinic in memory of their mother, who had died of cancer. It was the first clinic of its kind in the world.

The two researchers finally met Dr. L'Esperance, who greeted them cordially and showed them around the clinic. In the year after the clinic was started only forty-one patients went through. In its last eight months, in 1950, more than 2,000 were screened. During this time Dr. L'Esperance had established the validity and utility of the work of Georgios N. Papanicolaou, M.D., who became known as the father of modern cytology because of his outstanding contribution in the field of exfoliative cytology. Dr. Virginia was excited to meet him that day, and he eagerly showed Dr. Virginia some of his work. Dr. Virginia was careful to explain to me that today, it is thanks to his research that women are having their Pap smears regularly ("Pap" being the shortened form of his last name). She further explained that in a Pap smear the body cells that are cast off from the uterus, cervix, and vagina are scraped from the cervix, placed on a slide, and stained. Not only is the presence of cancer cells detected, but the amount of the body's estrogen is indicated by the size and shape of each cell's nucleus in relation to the cytoplasm. This test is also useful for determining the stage of menopause in women. Unfortunately, when the smear for cancer is positive, the cancer is already there. However, this test does permit early detection of some kinds of cancer of the female reproductive organs. The same method of cell determination is now applied to a number of other sites, such as lung and stomach. Until Dr. L'Esperance demonstrated the usefulness of the Pap smear at her cancer detection clinics, Dr. Papanicolaou's work had not been accepted in medical circles.

It was a thrill for Dr. Virginia to tell Dr. L'Esperance that she had found acid-fast organisms in all the tumors she had examined, and that they seemed to be similar to the ones she had observed in Hodgkin's disease. Dr. Virginia explained that she had cultured them, and that they were producing tumors in experimental animals. Dr. L'Esperance encouraged Dr. Virginia and Dr. Alexander-Jackson, and said she hoped they would have better success than she had had when she was doing her early work with Hodgkin's disease. Dr. L'Esperance then related the story of how she had isolated the acid-fast organisms from the glands of patients, made a culture, and then inoculated the organisms into guinea pigs. She reproduced the lesions and cultured the organisms again, fulfilling Koch's postulates. When she showed the animal tissues to James Ewing, M.D., the famous pathologist at the Cornell Medical Center, he confirmed the fact that the tissues were Hodgkin's disease. But when she told him that they were from experimentally inoculated guinea pigs, he suddenly changed his mind and insisted that they were not Hodgkin's disease, that it was impossible to reproduce the disease by cultures. Dr. L'Esperance was disgusted but continued with her work at the Strang Clinic until the technician she depended upon became ill. She was never able to replace her and retired soon after.

1 1

The Betrayal

What Dr. Virginia always referred to as a "betrayal" was actually a seminal event in the development of her theories into practical immunotherapy treatments. I once called it a "double-cross" but she rejected the term. In any event, it's the story of how the head of Memorial Sloan-Kettering Cancer Center in New York literally stole a $750,000 grant from her and subsequently drove her to the West Coast.

A Virus-Like Microorganism

During 1950, Dr. Virginia and her ally made many trips to Princeton, New Jersey, to take their filtered cultures to Dr. James Hillier at the RCA Victor Laboratories for electron microscopy. Dr. Hillier was very exacting in his studies of *P. cryptocides*. Many of the smaller bodies were beyond the range of the standard microscope. Repeated electron microscopic studies were made of pure microbic strains isolated from patients with cancer and scleroderma, and from chickens infected with the Rous "virus," or tumor agent. The filtered bodies appeared to be the same size as viruses. An electron photograph of the particles seen in mouse leukemia, and a similar one of the microbic structures they isolated in culture, illustrated the fact that the bodies in the mouse tissues and those Dr. Virginia cultured were undoubtedly the same agent. She felt that these studies definitely demonstrated that the so-called virus (or C-particles, or L-forms, or whatever name was currently in vogue) was the filterable form of her microbe, the hidden killer, *P. cryptocides*.

A Heat-Resistance Microorganism

Dr. Virginia and her associates exhibited their electron microscope work at a number of meetings and received great commendation, including, on one occasion, a prestigious Award of Merit. The cancer microbes were so tough and resistant to heat that at the lab's 1953 exhibit at the New York American Medical Association (AMA), the microbes stayed alive for five days while being televised around the exhibit by closed circuit set up by her friends at RCA. Visitors could watch the living bugs swimming about through the microscope on early black-and-white television; Dr. Virginia said it was the sensation of the exhibit. She expected great press coverage, but she claimed that, again, the formidable Dr. Cornelius Rhoads (profiled last chapter) forbade the New York AMA publicity people from interviewing her. She also said Dr. Rhoads threatened to withhold further news releases from the press if they reported on the findings of Dr. Virginia and her staff.

"They [the press] were intimidated by him and did not mention our exhibit at all, although there were crowds of people waiting to get into our booth," Dr. Virginia said. "Again, because of politics, we lost yet another chance to bring attention to our work."

A Transmissable Microorganism

Dr. Virginia and Dr. Alexander-Jackson had many other meetings of great interest to them. They visited the celebrated Dr. Peyton Rous at the Rockefeller Institute. This future Nobel laureate was very kindly and was interested in their work. They told him about growing the Rous agent in artificial media outside the living cell, and he said that he did not think this was unlikely or impossible.

(When he received the Nobel Prize for Medicine in 1966 at the age of eighty-seven, it was more than a half century since he had first reported the infectious nature of the chicken tumor that later bore his name.)

Dr. Virginia then met with Richard Shope, M.D., also of the Rockefeller Institute, who had identified the infectious agent of a rabbit tumor. On one occasion, at a meeting in Newark, Dr. Virginia had the temerity to differ with Dr. Shope on the type of cell in the Rous tumor that would transmit the cancer. Dr. Shope claimed that only the tumor cell could infect fresh chickens. Dr. Virginia insisted that this was not true, that any cell of the infected chicken could pass on the cancer, and that it need not be a cancer cell but only the *P. cryptocides* microbe in any seemingly normal cell from the infected host. In the case of blood, she insisted, the red blood cell itself could transmit the disease as well as any other cell, *whether cancerous or not*. To her, this was and remained an extremely important point, because whether a chicken displays a cancerous growth or not, many still contain the cancerous infectious agent within their bodies. (This is the reason she claimed it was not advisable for a cancer patient to eat poultry.) And if it was transmissible to the ape, she reasoned, it could be transmitted to a susceptible human being. However, Dr. Shope took issue with her contention, but promised to look up the information. To Dr. Virginia's great surprise, in a few days a generous letter of apology arrived, stating that her premise was correct and that he had been misinformed.

Another visit at that time was to the Lederle Laboratories in Pearl River, New York, where they became acquainted with Paul Little, who was in charge of Lederle's antitumor agent screening program. Mr. Little worked largely with the Rous sarcoma. At this point Lederle was excited about anti-folic agents, the folic-acid antagonists. Folic acid, a B vitamin, is the component processed by the liver that is essential for the prevention of pernicious anemia, a form of anemia that was considered fatal until the protective effects of the liver and, later, folic acid were discovered. At the time they were visiting Lederle Laboratories, it was felt that substances that substituted for and opposed folic acid could destroy tumors. These are called "analogs," derivatives or variants of the real vitamin made to "fool" the cancer cell in its requirement for the essential vitamin; the cancer incorporates the analog into the cell and is killed. Dr. Virginia called it a kind of "nutritional Trojan horse."

In 1948, Sidney Farber, M.D., of Children's Hospital in Boston initiated the era of analogs in cancer research by injecting some children with a drug called aminopterin, after which they showed a remarkable return to health. Unfortunately, the recovery was only temporary; at best a few lived up to a year or two. Aminopterin is still in use today. Farber's minor success touched off a search for analogs, false vitamins, false hormones, and other chemical agents. However, Dr. Virginia was not impressed, because, she said, even though chickens previously infected with Rous sarcoma and then given Dr. Farber's analog did not develop tumors, they either died of folic-acid deprivation or of other forms of the Rous disease. She warned Mr. Little during the meeting that her bacterial cultures of the Rous-infected chickens treated with the folic-acid antagonists showed no diminution in the amount of growth of the causative agent. There were numerous round-table discussions with the staff at Lederle. Although conducted in a congenial atmosphere, the conversations always ended in a "stalemate," as Dr. Virginia put it. She couldn't agree with them, but they insisted that a bacterial culture from a so-called virus-induced tumor, such as Rous sarcoma, was impossible.

A Tumor-Causing Microorganism

On another occasion, they went to the Bronx Botanical Gardens to request some cultures of *Bacterium tumefaciens* (*Agrobacterium tumefaciens*). Dr. Virginia's interest there was because of the discovery of *Bacterium tumefaciens* by Erwin F. Smith, Ph.D., in January 1908, and his report of his production of malignant growth in plants with this microorganism in the April 1916 issue of the *Journal of Cancer Research*. (Dr. Virginia's near-photographic memory constantly astonished me.) Dr. Smith was then a noted pathologist in charge of the laboratory of plant pathology for the U.S. Department of Agriculture. He was also a bacteriologist and a former president of the Society of American Bacteriologists. He produced cancers in plants at will by injections of *Bacterium tumefaciens*. In plants these tumors are called "crown galls." The diseased plants can be seen anywhere in the United States if one just knows what to look for. A number of investigators thought that *Bacterium tumefaciens* could produce cancers in animals and perhaps even in humans. The work of Erwin F. Smith had a profound influence on Charles Mayo, M.D., of the famed Mayo Clinic, who reported on October 28, 1925, at an American College of Surgeons meeting:

> Down in Washington, in the government laboratories of the Department of Agriculture, Erwin Smith, a very well-known government bacteriologist, is carrying on a most interesting series of experiments on plants. He has rows on rows of plants in which he has been able to transplant cancer, resembling the disease in human beings. So exact are his experiments that he is able to foretell with absolute accuracy just how long it will require the cancerous growth to break out on the plant stock, and more than that, just where it will break out.

At the Bronx Botanical Gardens, Dr. Virginia was given a tube of the living microbes and admonished not to drop the bottle, because she held in her hands enough microbes to infect half the state of New York. Dr. Alexander-Jackson held the bottle very securely while Dr. Virginia drove back to the Newark laboratory. There, they observed the microbes in culture and then injected a living culture into mice. With large doses, the mice died overnight; with small doses, they lived longer. Franz Gerlach, Ph.D., who was at the laboratory at the time, thought that on gross examination the diseased tissues resembled sarcomas. However, they didn't pursue this study any further except to note that the culture was pathogenic for mice on injection. (At the time of our meeting, Dr. Virginia showed me electron microphotographs of the culture that she had kept through the years.) The organism appeared to be endemic in the soil, but they thought it could also be transmitted by an insect vector (a carrier that transmits disease). There was a young peach tree in the backyard that appeared healthy and sported pretty blossoms in spring. However, several of the peaches that ripened on it had tumorous swellings on them. On staining these tumors she found bacilli. Dr. Virginia warned her husband not to eat the peaches and to cut down the tree and burn it. (She always felt that all trees and vegetation bearing the crown gall should be destroyed by burning and the underlying soil sterilized, if possible.)

A Cell-Penetrating, Cancer-Causing Microorganism

Just prior to our meeting in La Jolla, an exciting article appeared in *Scientific American*, June 1983, entitled "A Vector for Introducing New Genes into Plants." It described how a bacterium, *A. tumefaciens*, can insert a piece of its DNA into a healthy plant cell, causing a genetic modification in the plant cell that turned it into a cancer cell, and which then multiplied into a full tumor called crown gall tumor. The mechanism of this transformation was fully explained in the article. No virus was implicated. Dr. Virginia took great joy in the article because, as she reasoned, "If a bacterium can transform a healthy cell of a plant into a plant cancer, is it not logical to suppose a human bacterium could transform a healthy human cell into a human cancer without any implication of a virus?"

Dr. Virginia claimed there is a marked similarity in the way *P. cryptocides* evolves a genome to produce human choriogonadotropin (HCG) in the cell. She said the major difference is that *P. cryptocides* is latent (inactive) in the normal cell and becomes actively, producing HCG, under certain conditions.

Of her many associations, Dr. Virginia considered her visits with

Drs. Irene and William Diller of Philadelphia to have been the most rewarding and enjoyable. Dr. Irene Diller, then editor of the biological journal *Growth,* was associated with the Institute for Cancer Research in Philadelphia. She was not only a famous research scientist in the field of animal tumors but also a linguist, an interpreter at scientific meetings, a scientific librarian, a cytologist, and an authority on chemotherapeutic agents and their effects on tumorous and normal animal tissues. She was especially interested in the relationship of microorganisms to cancerous tissues. Dr. Diller had always been a fount of information concerning research in other countries. She kept the Newark researchers abreast of much of the foreign literature. At a scientific meeting in 1953, her paper entitled, "Studies of Fungoidal Forms Found in Malignancy" discussed fungoidal forms found as contaminants in animal tumors and other types of organisms that seemed to have a more specific relationship to cancer. At that time, Dr. Diller had not worked with the mycobacterium-like microbe that Dr. Virginia was later to designate as *Progenitor cryptocides.* In later years, after she began to work with the same type of microbes that Dr. Virginia was isolating, she did monumental work in fulfilling Koch's postulates with her isolates by increasing production of tumors in mice of known spontaneous tumor incidence.

Dr. Diller also demonstrated by her blood-culture method that, of fifty-six mice that became tumor-bearing during their lifetime, forty-nine (93 percent) were carrying the organism in their blood by one year of age. In 1,400 additional mice studied by this method, a very high correlation was established between the presence of the organisms in the blood and the eventual production of tumors.

Dr. Diller also catalyzed Dr. Virginia's association with other scientists in the cancer field because of her wide range of acquaintances through her editorship of *Growth,* as well as other worldwide contacts. Her work was, in general, confirmatory of Dr. Virginia's, and she made many additional contributions to the work at the Newark lab.

A Microbe Refuted

Now comes the betrayal. Dr. Virginia always blamed "the long polit-ical arm" of Dr. Cornelius P. Rhoads for the closing of the Newark laboratory. On April 10, 1951, the *Newark Evening News* announced that $750,000 in cancer research funds had been given to the Pres-byterian Hospital in Newark. (A small fortune in those days.) The same amount was given to the Memorial Sloan-Kettering Cancer Center in New York, which Dr. Rhoads headed. In announcing the grants, the trustees expressed the hope that Presbyterian Hospital in years to come would develop into a leading cancer center. The foundation was set in the estates of two South Orange, New Jersey, sisters named Black. The accumulated residuary estate of $1,500,000 was left in trust "for the charitable purpose of providing treatment and care both preventive and remedial, for needy persons who may be afflicted or threatened with the disease of cancer." The bequest stemmed from the tragic death from cancer of the husband of one of the Black sisters, John A. Black, in 1921, only two years after their marriage. It also specified that the funds go to an institution in New Jersey or in New York. There was a five-year deadline for the dis-bursement of the funds. Another Mr. Black, the brother of the deceased, went to the publisher of the *Newark Evening News,* to make an appeal for help, and the paper then ran the column asking for suggestions.

More than 5,000 replies were sent in. The trustees, after much deliberation, decided that Presbyterian Hospital and Memorial Sloan-Kettering best met the conditions of the estate. In discussing the gift to Presbyterian, the trustees said that "although it is a general hospital as contrasted to the reputation of Memorial [Sloan Kettering] Center as the best-known cancer institute in the world, Presbyterian's personnel and associations are adaptable to a degree of specialization in the treatment and prevention of cancer. Presby-terian conducts a cancer clinic and a speech clinic for laryngecto-mized patients. Cooperative research activities on cancer supported by grants from the Damon Runyon Fund, Abbott Laboratories, and the American Cancer Society are being conducted on the premises by the Presbyterian branch of Rutgers University Bureau of Biological Research." Officials of the two hospitals then gave written agreements pledging faith with the vision of the Black sisters for helping cancer victims. Dr. Virginia, affiliated with the Presbyterian Hospital, was not to know how that faith was betrayed for more than a year.

In the meantime, she was conducting her animal immunization programs, exhibiting at numerous medical and scientific meetings, and preparing her material for presentation at the Sixth International Congress of Microbiology in Rome. After exhibiting at the American Medical Association Conference in June 1953, she left on August 5 for Europe.

She and her team were received with much cordiality on their arrival in London. There, they presented their papers and discussed them with colleagues who would be participating in the upcoming Rome congress. Dr. Virginia was particularly interested in meeting with Dr. Emmy Klieneberger-Nobel at the Lister Institute. Dr. Klieneberger-Nobel was the scientist who first described L-forms of bacteria, which are bacterial forms without cell walls. (She called them L-forms for Lister Institute, where she was doing her research.)

While Dr. Virginia was in London she also spent a day with Dr. Ernest Brieger of the Strangeways Laboratory at Cambridge University. He had worked both in England and in the United States on the filterable forms of the tubercle bacillus, using electron microscopy techniques. A number of previous investigators had described a complex life cycle for the tubercle bacillus, among them Dr. Leon Grigoraki. However, Dr. Grigoraki did not carry the work to the filter-passing stage, nor did he have the electron microscope to demonstrate how the organisms were invisible under the light microscope.

The team then flew from London to Frankfurt, Germany, the nearest air terminal to Bad Kreuznach, where they planned to visit Dr. Wilhelm von Brehmer, who had worked with the same microorganism Dr. Virginia was calling *P. cryptocides*. (Of course, he called it by another name, *Syphonospora polymorpha von Brehmer.*)

The Sixth International Congress of Microbiology took place in Rome from September 6 to 12. Scientists arrived from all over the world, representing many fields of microbiological research. Two Nobel Prize winners, Sir Alexander Fleming (penicillin) and Dr. Selman Waksman (streptomycin, and the man who coined the word "antibiotic"), were present, and Dr. Virginia eagerly discussed her work with them.

On the afternoon of September 9, the little-known group from the Presbyterian Hospital of Newark, New Jersey, presented their papers. Even almost thirty years later, there was excitement in Dr. Virginia's voice as she told me that these papers presented incontrovertible proof of the presence of the *P. cryptocides* in tissues, their cultural properties, their identification as specific microorganisms, and their ability to produce pathogenic lesions in experimental animals. They also demonstrated that immune bodies can be produced that indicate the close relationship of these organisms to one another, whether of human or animal strains, and that the so-called viruses of animal tumors could well be the filterable forms of these causative bacteria. In addition, these microorganisms could produce immune bodies that affect the course of the disease in the infected host.

The total presentation of Dr. Virginia's team was nothing less than sensational. The reportage in the scientific and general press was worldwide.

The team was not aware, though, that the coverage by the *New York Times*, the *Washington Post*, and their own hometown newspapers would incite the wrath of American scientists. Upon their return, they were met on the dock by several newspaper science reporters who told Dr. Virginia that the papers presented in Rome were being challenged.

Here is an example of one article from Dr. Virginia's scrapbook:

"New York Doctors Challenge Cancer Germ Report"

A spokesman for the New York Academy of Medicine today discounted claims of a medical research team that a cancer-causing microorganism has been isolated and that it has yielded an anti-cancer serum in animals. The spokesman, Dr. Iago Galdston, executive secretary of the academy's Committee on Medical Information, said the presence of germs in cancerous tissue has been noted before, but these appear to move in after the cancer has developed.

"This is an old story and it has not stood up under investigation," he said. "Microorganisms found in malignant tumors have been found to be secondary invaders and not the primary cause of the malignancy."

The claim was made yesterday in Rome at the Sixth International Congress of Microbiology by a New Jersey research team. They pictured cancer as a generalized disease caused by an organism in the human bloodstream, and reported that rabbits and sheep inoculated with an antiserum produced "potent immune bodies." Members of the team were Dr. Virginia Wuerthele-Caspe, Dr. Eleanor Alexander-Jackson, Dr. L. W. Smith and Dr. G. A. Clark, all associated with Presbyterian Hospital in Newark. (Pers. comm., 1983)

Dr. Virginia said she had expected a refutation of her work, of course, since in 1953 it was felt that cancer was not an infectious process but a metabolic or deficiency disease. (The complex cycle has come full circle again, so that today almost every scientist believes that cancer is an infection but that no specific agent has yet been identified. It was not until her classification at the 1969 New York Academy of Science meetings that she was able to present the full scope of her work to the American scientific world.) However, the 1953 newspaper refutations were for the most part inaccurate and merely echoed a lot of the establishment questioning she had been getting all along.

Upon their eventual return to the laboratory, though, they were still exhilarated by their successes in Europe and the recognition received from world-renowned scientific giants. Dr. Virginia was convinced that when she got the upcoming share of the $750,000 grant she would finally be able to proceed with the work that would eventually lead to a completely new attitude toward the treatment of cancer, and perhaps even develop a vaccine for its cure.

However, she was met with the cruel reality of what had transpired behind her back. Dr. Virginia believed that as a man named Hardin, one of the directors of the Black grant, lay dying of cancer at Sloan-Kettering, he had been prevailed upon to sign a codicil to the Black bequest, stating that the researchers at Presbyterian Hospital could not spend their share of the grant without the permission of Dr. Rhoads at Sloan-Kettering. And as it turned out, the only acquisitions Dr. Rhoads would allow Dr. Virginia were a new wing to be added to the hospital and the installation of a high-voltage cobalt radiation machine that he had already purchased!

Dr. Virginia was enraged. She considered that the sisters Black were betrayed, as well as were her and Dr. Alexander-Jackson, who had labored so long and diligently to establish a top-flight research laboratory devoted to the *biological* approach to the treatment of cancer, and *not* to radiation. Moreover, Dr. Virginia always claimed that it was her team's work that brought the $750,000 gift to Presbyterian in the first place, yet it was the radiation machine this gift purchased that destroyed all she had accomplished.

At the time of the announcement of the Black grant, Dr. Virginia had been elated. She could foresee establishing preventive clinics across the nation that would screen patients and immunize them when they were bacteriologically positive; clinics that would promote better life habits, better nutrition, safer and cleaner surroundings, industrial and environmental control of carcinogens, earlier detection of precancerous lesions, and genetic counseling.

It was a great dream while it lasted.

12

San Diego:
The Last Stop

Knowing Dr. Virginia's personality and temperament at the time, I could imagine her launching into a rage when she heard her grant money had been used to buy a radiation machine. Although I never heard her use profanity, I could imagine the epithets hurled in the direction of Dr. Cornelius Rhoads's office at Memorial Sloan-Kettering Cancer Center across the river. But as she told me the story sitting on her couch in the La Jolla mansion, she was quiet and a little teary-eyed as she recalled the moment she decided to leave New Jersey.

Dr. Virginia considered the ten years in Newark to be the most productive years of her life, and it was with great sadness that she realized it had come to an end. She said she thought of all the babies she had delivered, the many wounds she had sewn up, the patients she had treated and healed, the students and teachers she had met and befriended, the clinics she had attended, the many cancer patients she had cared for . . . and above all, the laboratory in which she and her colleagues had toiled so tirelessly, with such high hopes and ambitions, now dismantled and never to be opened again.

Perhaps when cancer is stamped out for good, she told me, just like polio and smallpox, the world will know that much of the pioneering work started in that innovative little laboratory in Newark.

She consoled herself with the thought that she was going to join her family in California; her parents and her sister lived there. It was 1953. She and her husband bought a house in Beverly Hills. She became an active member of the Los Angeles (LA) County Medical Society, but she couldn't find a research position and had to content herself with work in the LA Board of Education's general medical office at the Civic Center. The work was interesting, but life on the LA freeways got her down and they eventually moved to San Diego where she began work at the San Diego Health Association Clinic as a medical internist and clinician. It was at that time that her current husband, Dr. Joseph Caspe, died of diabetes and heart disease. She was now almost fifty years old, a widow, 3,000 miles from her pioneering work in Newark, New Jersey, and beginning a totally new life.

The new life was busy indeed. As the only woman at the San Diego clinic and the last physician hired (female doctors were still rare at the time), she worked almost double-time to become accepted by the rest of the staff and to establish her name in the area, as well as to keep her eye open for research opportunities. It was at the clinic that she met A. M. Livingston, M.D., who was head of the Eye, Ear, Nose, Throat, and Allergy Department, and, a few years later, in 1957, they were married. (This was apparently the great love of her life, as she frequently spoke adoringly of Dr. Livingston, even in the presence of her forbearing subsequent husband, Dr. Owen Wheeler.)

Medical Orthodoxy Begins to Catch Up

Although she was no longer actively engaged in cancer research, except in the clinical aspect of cancer detection, her papers from the Rome congress had sparked a great deal of interest among several distinguished European scientists who believed in the infectious nature of cancer. They, too, had isolated the pleomorphic microorganism that she called *P. cryptocides*. Though they were calling it by a number of different names, what they saw was undoubtedly some form of the same causative agent. Dr. Virginia had no quarrel with the European investigators. (In fact, I never heard a hint of professional jealousy when she discussed the research of others.) She believed she was the first investigator to show that the causative organism was an Actinomycetales, which includes the tubercle bacillus, and that the so-called viruses of animal tumors were, in reality, filterable forms of this same organism. Dr. Alexander-Jackson's work in the pleomorphism of the lepra and tubercle bacilli greatly enhanced this concept.

Dr. Alexander-Jackson had become interested in the European group and was appointed the American secretary to the First International Congress for Microbiology of Cancer and Leukemia. A congress was set up in Antwerp, and Dr. Virginia was named one of three vice-presidents. Dr. E. Villequez, director of the Central Blood Bank of France and professor of experimental medicine at the University of Dijon, France, was the president. The other vice presidents were Drs. F. Gerlach from the University of Vienna, Austria, and Clara J. Fonti, president of the Centro Internazionale Oncological di Viggio, Milan, Italy.

On Monday, July 14, 1958, the congress convened. The opening began with an address by the president on "Humanism and the Struggle Against Cancer." Dr. Virginia had the honor of being the first speaker of the scientific session. The papers presented were entirely concerned with the immunological approach to the cancer problem. Dr. Virginia considered this material to be far in advance of the work being done in the United States. The example she gave me was the work of Dr. Robert Huebner of the National Cancer Institute's division of virology, who proposed his theory of the C-particle, a noncontagious virus, to be the cause of cancer when activated. This Huebner theory, on which great sums of money would eventually be expended, was old hat at the time it was proposed because it had already been presented in Europe.

At the afternoon meeting of the congress, Dr. Nello Mori, director of the Instituto Microbiologicol Bella Vista, Naples, Italy spoke on "My Conception of the Causative-Pathological Symbiosis of a Certain Parasite in Cancer and Methods of Combating the Parasite by Immunization." Dr. Gerlach spoke on "Latency and Regression of Tumors Brought About by Specific Therapy." Dr. Clara Fonti spoke on the "Pathogenic Etiology of Cancer and Its Treatment." Dr. Eleanor Alexander-Jackson showed her film on the "Morphological Changes in the Human Tubercle Bacillus." Dr. Irene Diller spoke on the "Morphological Changes in Mouse and Rat Blood."

Dr. Virginia said that in 1958 all these distinguished scientists had been carrying on significant research in the biological and immunological treatment of cancer for years. And when we started to prepare her book in 1983, she said the United States orthodoxy was only then beginning to catch up. She alleged that "suppressive" actions of the American Cancer Society, the American Medical Association, and the Food and Drug Administration severely retarded the progress of American scientists. She further alleged that the deliberate suppression of some work in this country had set cancer research back a number of decades. She stated,

> If the animal immunization studies done by Shope and others in this country had been regarded as prototypes for human immunization, and the early work of Glover, Gregory, and L'Esperance had been taken more seriously, cancer treatment would now be far advanced. This work has been ignored because certain powerful individuals backed by large monetary grants can become the dictators of research and suppress all work that does not promote their interests or that may present a threat to their prestige.

Of particular interest to Dr. Virginia at the congress was the work of Dr. Clara Fonti. In the autumn of 1958, Dr. Fonti wrote a book entitled *Eziopatogenesi del Cancro* (*Etiology and Pathogenesis of Cancer*), published by Amedeo Nicola & Co., in Milan. The book revealed that she had developed a method of staining preserved blood slides so that the presence of the cancer infection could be evaluated in the blood of patients. Her procedures and treatments were thoroughly documented in the book. It was painstakingly written with great accuracy and had many beautiful color illustrations. What impressed Dr. Virginia above all was Chapter 3 on *Autocontagio,* or self-infection. Dr. Fonti had inoculated the skin on her chest between her breasts with a cancer culture—not with the cells but with the culture. When a cancerous growth developed in the area, Dr. Fonti removed it and had it analyzed. The diagnosis revealed that the cancer had been produced through the inoculation of a *bacterial culture.* There was a photograph of the lesion as well as a photomicrograph of the pathological section with the diagnosis of a "basal cell epithelioma." Dr. Virginia said anyone who had studied the microbiology of cancer became convinced by Dr. Fonti's experiment that the disease is infectious but not contagious; that is, that it can only be transmitted by direct contact.

Soon after she returned to the United States, a heavy workload resumed again. Both Dr. Virginia and her husband worked long hours at the clinic. It was during this period that Dr. Virginia suffered a near fatal heart attack and had to curtail her medical activities for a few years while she recuperated.

An Immunological Approach to Cancer

During the recuperation, Dr. Alexander-Jackson received a grant from the National Institutes of Health (NIH) to continue with the Rous work at the Institute of Comparative Medicine at the College of Physicians and Surgeons of Columbia University in New York. Meanwhile, Dr. Irene Diller and her colleagues at the Institute for Cancer Research in Philadelphia were carrying on corroborative studies of the acid-fast organisms Dr. Virginia had first discovered back in 1947. In March 1965, Dr. Diller was invited to New Orleans to attend the annual American Cancer Society (ACS) seminar for science writers. True to character, Irene gave a fair and impartial presentation of the microbiological approaches to the cancer problem in which they had all collaborated. Dr. Virginia read about the report in the *San Diego Union*. As a result of Irene's presentation, Dr. Virginia and Dr. Alexander-Jackson were invited to present papers at the next ACS science writers seminar that was held the following March in Phoenix, Arizona. (These seminars had been initiated by Patrick McGrady Sr. as a means of telling the tax-paying, gift-donating public what was being done with the money invested in cancer research.) The invitation Dr. Virginia received was signed by Dr. Harold S. Diehl, senior vice president for research and medical affairs of the ACS. She also knew that her old friend Patrick McGrady Sr. would be in charge of the science writers and their scheduled releases. It was considered a great honor to be invited to become a member of the faculty of the seminar, because thereafter the names of the participants were kept permanently on the faculty roster. McGrady told her that he'd scheduled them for the last day of the program since their material was considered controversial, and he thought there would be less commotion after their presentations at that time.

She thought the timing of the presentation was wise. Whenever anyone presents a new concept and criticizes the old ones, the presenter must be prepared to stand the "slings and arrows" (her term, quoting Shakespeare) that invariably follow. Dr. Virginia knew what would happen when she and her colleague stood on the podium and presented their papers. She was proposing new methods of immunological treatment of cancer in humans. She told me she felt like the bull's-eye in the target of a dart game.

Before mounting the podium she took the opportunity of slipping away to the ladies' room where she fortified herself with a mild sedative and a heart pill. Then she offered up a silent prayer that there would be ears to hear and minds and hearts that would open to her message.

She had intended only to present the theoretical aspects of determining the cancer-prone individual and to suggest future methods for preventive immunization. Also, she wanted to convince the knowledgeable audience that cancer is an infection, and that surgery, radiation, and chemicals cannot eradicate a continuing infectious process. She stated that a "screening program of the entire population could be undertaken by routine blood cultures to determine the presence of these mycobacteria, correlated with evaluation of blood smears and related to immune competency by various methods of antigen-antibody determination." Both she and Dr. Alexander-Jackson claimed that this organism had the ability to change its form and might vary its appearance from that of a fungus to that of a cluster of virus-sized pleuro-pneumonia-like organisms (PPLO), or mycoplasma. She did not intend at that time to discuss some of her earliest efforts in immunizing patients. But when she was asked if that were possible, she replied that it was and cited three early cases. Immediately (and typically), the press misquoted her and the following day's headlines blared that she claimed she had a "cure for cancer" by immunization, even though that was not their main objective in the presentation of their work. In the original presentation, she stated that the collagenic mycobacteria, which include the cancer organism, have thrown researchers off for years because they are able to change their forms. She also reported that, in a series of breast-cancer studies at the Naval Hospital in San Diego, the best results were obtained with surgery alone, the next best with surgery and radiation, and the worst with surgery, radiation, and chemicals.

Dr. Virginia went on to imply that the cobalt machine might reduce the size of the tumors but contributed very little to the long-term cure of the disease. Dr. John Lawrence of the Lawrence Radiation Laboratories (now called the Lawrence Livermore Laboratories) had previously stated that his hope was for a cobalt machine in every town and village in the United States. Typical of Dr. Virginia, when she heard that statement she began to wave a petri dish (used for making cultures) over her head and shouting at the podium that it could be mightier than all the high-powered radiation machines in the world. The tactful Dr. Diehl tried to smooth over the commotion by stating, "Thousands of patients have been cured by surgery and radiation, but, of course, we hope that research will eventually render these treatments unnecessary."

Medical Orthodoxy Begins to Open Up

The Phoenix newspapers were kind. One reported the "basic requirements for formation of the cancer cell to be the causative microorganism and that all other factors such as coal-tar irritants, other microorganisms, the aging process, any chronic irritants leading to poor local resistance and giving rise to immature, susceptible reparative cells may prepare the soil for the multiplication of the cancer organism and its penetration into the cytoplasm and nucleus of the host." Patrick McGrady said, "It could be they are right. Cynicism has never cured cancer and never will." Dr. Jorgen Fogh, a virologist at Memorial Sloan-Kettering Cancer Center , said in an interview that he had examined more than 150 cancers, including a dozen leukemias, and had found nothing that resembled mycoplasma or the PPLO.

Meanwhile, Dr. Leon Dmoschowski of the University of Texas–MD Anderson Hospital and Tumor Institute was coming up with evidence that mycoplasma may, indeed, play a part in cancer. This was reported widely, and it seemed to Dr. Virginia that the point of view favored depends on the prestige of the institution rather than on the merits of the research.

Three years later, in the *Journal of the American Medical Association,* July 28, 1969, there was a summary of the work of K. A. Bisset, who wrote in the *New Scientist,* June 12, 1969, that "Various mycoplasmas have been suspected of causing some disease whose etiology is not yet clear." He speculated that many diseases could be caused by mycoplasmas or by parts of this elusive bacterium. "The fact that mycoplasmas can break down into virus-like particles, easily identifiable on electron-microscope examination and similar to those found in the blood of leukemia patients, leads to a strong suspicion that mycoplasma may be a culprit in the development of certain malignant processes." Also, Dr. Bernard Roswit, reporting in Chicago at the Radiological Society of North America on the year-long study of more than 500 patients at seventeen Veterans' Administration (VA) hospitals, had recently stated, "At present it appears that the patient is at the mercy of his cancer and his survival depends more upon the stage of the disease, type of cell, and biological character of the cancer than upon the therapeutic act."

The patients in the VA study were divided into two groups with half receiving the best of radiation treatment and the other half only sugar pills. At the end of the year only 18 percent of the radiated were alive, while 14 percent of those getting sugar pills alone survived. Those treated lived only 30 days longer than the untreated, and none of the patients in either group was cured. However, Dr. Roswit said the radiation did shrink the tumors temporarily and helped the morale of the patients, but it did not prolong life.

It was one of Dr. Virginia's pet theories that a general "uniformity of conformity" is being forced upon the American public. A doctor who does not conform can lose hospital privileges. If the patient does not conform, insurance carriers may refuse to pay the insurance. And so on. She asked, "Does not each individual have the right to decide what may be done to his or her body? In some hospitals, patients have been put on double-blind studies in which neither they nor their physicians know what treatments they are getting. In certain cases cancer victims have been forced to wear wigs so that no one will know whether a drug is causing their baldness. They are herded like sheep into pens for medical treatment about which they are neither informed nor consulted."

The First Human Patient

For the three recuperative years following her heart attack in 1962, Dr. Virginia was relatively inactive in cancer research but was giv-

ing a lot of thought to her future. The seeds of independence were
starting to grow once more, and her restlessness added to the begin-
nings of the idea of opening up her own immunotherapy clinic. She
devoted most of her time in that period to teaching mental health
and hygiene and to community volunteer work with the San Diego
Symphony, the Children's Adoption Society, the Opera Guild, the
local Vassar Alumnae Association, the La Jolla Pen Women, and others. During this time something happened which, although she did-
n't realize it at the time, was probably the event that ultimately
resulted in the writing of her book (and this one, for that matter).

When she was in the hospital, a close friend who had been bringing care packages to her on a regular basis appeared one day with
sad news. The friend's husband, a physician, had a malignant tumor
of the thymus gland, which along with the heart and major blood
vessels, is located in the middle of the chest cavity. His lymphoma
was diagnosed as being bigger than a baseball. An operation
revealed that there was nothing that could be done, since the tumor
had grown into all the surrounding tissues and couldn't be removed. His doctors said that radiation might be temporarily help-
ful, but were honest in telling him that no one seriously thought he
could be helped for long. (Dr. Virginia recalled making a mental note
of a serious car accident he had had a few years earlier that had
required large amounts of blood from the local blood bank.)

While telling Dr. Virginia about her husband, the friend broke
down in tears. Then she blurted, "Oh, Dr. Virginia! You know so
much about cancer, and you are always talking so proudly about
how you're saving animals from tumors! Can't you do the same
thing for my husband? Can't you do *anything* for Ralph?" Dr. Virginia was reluctant to undertake treating him, but they were both
such dear friends that she agreed to take a look at him.

When she got out of the hospital, the ailing friend became her
first human patient.

She treated him with an autogenous vaccine as a nonspecific
immune stimulation, mild antibiotics, and diet. At the time I inter-

viewed her, he had died only recently, of a heart attack, after living almost twenty additional years. (For recent developments on cancer vaccines, see "News Update: Autogenous Vaccines Are Here," below.)

NEWS UPDATE: AUTOGENOUS VACCINES ARE HERE!

When Dr. Virginia mentioned her autogenous vaccines and described how she made patients' vaccines from their own tumors, the medical community rolled its collective eyes and dismissed her as a quack. A cancer vaccine? Preposterous. Yet, today, vaccines for cancer treatment are being studied at hundreds of laboratories around the world. If you google "Cancer and Vaccines" at ClinicalTrials.gov, you'll see more than 1,000 studies presented. Some of them show dramatic promise and are being described by many of our most important and revered institutions. To cite just a few:

- In 2011, the Food and Drug Administration (FDA) approved a drug called ipilimumab (Yervoy), or "ippy" for short, developed by Dr. James Allison at the MD Anderson Cancer Center in Houston. The drug is now being manufactured for the treatment of melanoma. According to an April 16, 2014, story in the *Houston Chronicle,* Dr. Allison is credited with "one of the most important breakthroughs in cancer history." The president of MD Anderson, Dr. Ron DePinho, thinks Dr. Allison will win the Nobel Prize. He said, "By creating this brilliant approach that treats the immune system rather than the tumor, Jim Allison opened a completely new avenue for treating cancers that's the most exciting and promising area of cancer research today." A Nobel Prize for treating the immune system? Where have we heard that before?

- In 2010, the first prostate cancer vaccine, called sipuleucel (Provenge), was approved by the FDA. An autogenous vaccine, Provenge works by removing white blood cells (immune cells) from the patient, exposing them to a certain protein that serves as a marker, and then re-injecting the cells into the patient. This triggers the patient's own immune system to start attacking and killing the prostate cancer cells.

- In 2008, the FDA approved two autogenous vaccines, Gardasil and Cervarix, that protect against 70 percent of all cases of cervical cancer, according to the National Cancer Institute (NCI). The vaccines were developed in parallel studies at Georgetown University Medical Center, the University of Rochester, the University of Queensland, Australia, and the NCI. Gardasil is a prophylactic vaccine that prevents human papillomavirus (HPV) infections but that doesn't work *after* the infection sets in. Hence, the FDA recommends vaccination before adolescence and the onset of sexual activity. Cervarix works similarly to Gardasil. Both were developed at about the same time.

In addition, many vaccines are in late-stage test programs and are nearing completion with the next step being submission to the FDA for approval of a commercial product. Here are several among them:

- In 2000, scientists at the Dana Farber Cancer Institute at Harvard Medical School, in conjunction with the University of Goettingen, Germany, announced the development of an autogenous vaccine made from patients' tumors and dendritic cells (blood cells that trap foreign material) to boost immune systems and reduce tumors. Dr. Donald W. Kufe at Dana Farber was quoted as saying, "On x-rays and scans you can actually see (the tumors) go away." After 75 patients with highly metastasized kidney and skin cancers were vaccinated, they saw their tumors "melt away within weeks," according to a *Harvard Gazette* article at the time. The patients had no side effects and the tumors remained absent two and three years later. Kufe's team also successfully treated patients with metastatic breast and prostate cancer. In Germany, co-researchers were getting similar "amazing" results with lung and brain tumors. In a 2010 issue of the *Journal of the American Society of Hematology*, Kufe and his colleagues announced the development of a vaccine for multiple myeloma.

- In 2012, after the NCI tested an autogenous vaccine for boosting the immune system of non-Hodgkin's lymphoma patients and licensed it to a biopharmaceutical company to develop into a commercial product, the FDA began testing it. The vaccine, called BiovaxID, is in Phase 3 (late-stage) testing.

- At Johns Hopkins' Sol Goldman Pancreatic Cancer Research Center, scientists are zeroing in on an autogenous vaccine to treat pancreatic cancer. The vaccine only works for patients who have been specifically diagnosed with pancreatic cancer and energizes the immune system to attack the cancer cells.

- An ongoing immunologic study, begun in 2013 at the University of Pittsburgh School of Medicine, is investigating an autogenous vaccine for pancreatic and colorectal cancers based on a mucin molecule called mucine-1 (MUC1). The vaccine is being used on patients who have shown by colonoscopy to have recurrent polyps.

- At Memorial Sloan-Kettering, Dr. Lloyd Old, one of the pioneers of treating bladder cancer with BCG, said before his death in 2011, "We are entering a new era in the development of cancer vaccines. We have identified key antigens for constructing vaccines, and we are beginning to learn how to put them together." Dr. Robert Maki, also of Sloan–Kettering, conducted a study several years ago in which ten patients with pancreatic cancer were given an autogenous vaccine from a heat-shock protein (an abundant molecule present in all cells). The patients had a median survival of 2.5 years, whereas the average survival after surgery for pancreatic cancer is 14 to 15 months. Maki reported that one patient was still without disease after five years and that two other patients were disease-free after more than two years following treatment. "This heat-shock-protein-based cancer vaccine contains the antigenic fingerprint of the patient's particular cancer, and is designed to direct the body's immune system to target and destroy only cancer cells bearing that specific antigenic fingerprint," Dr. Maki said.

The work on vaccines goes on and on, and is exciting indeed. All kinds of cancers, with major emphasis on colorectal and pancreatic cancer vaccines, are being tested with promising immunologic results. All this is happening only a single generation after Dr. Virginia Livingston-Wheeler, the true pioneer in autogenous cancer vaccines, was reviled for her immunologic therapies.

The friend's husband was so pleased with his recovery that he put Dr. Virginia in touch with a friend of his, another physician in San Diego, with whom she then collaborated on treating the immune systems of a few of his patients, with excellent results. Finally, the friend asked one of his wealthier patients to give Dr. Virginia a grant so that she could continue some of her research. That small grant was then followed by a grant from the Fleet Foundation of San Diego, which continued for several years. Later on, the Fleet grant formed the nucleus of the Livingston Fund at the University of California, San Diego (UCSD), which then moved to the Livingston-Wheeler Medical Clinic. Gifts from patients and friends also kept her research work going.

In order to receive the Fleet grant, Dr. Virginia had to affiliate with a nonprofit group, so that money could be donated tax-free. She chose the San Diego Biomedical Group, an association of scientists consisting of physicians, engineers, and college professors, and she set up a small lab at the Biomedical Institute, where she worked for a year. Simultaneously, she also opened a small office in the neighborhood, which allowed her to consult with a few patients on a research basis. Dr. Eleanor Alexander-Jackson came out to stay with her for a month, and they again went over the work she was doing to reconfirm the presence and cultural properties of the *P. cryptocides* group. Eventually, when her technician left on maternity leave, she decided she needed larger facilities, so she joined UCSD as associate professor of microbiology.

By the summer of 1968 she had gravitated to what would eventually become the Livingston Medical Clinic. Dr. Alexander-Jackson came out again to stay with her for three months, and in addition to her husband, she had a full-time technician, a medical student, and Dr. Gerhard Wolter from San Diego State College (SDSU) working together with them in the UCSD laboratory. They carried on extensive bacteriological work on *P. cryptocides,* which led to the "landmark" group of papers presented at the 1969 meeting of the New York Academy of Sciences, where they formally presented the classification of the cancer-causing microbe.

Dr. Alexander-Jackson acted as chairman for their section, which was called "Microorganisms Associated with Malignancy." For the record, and for readers who may wish to review these papers for technical reasons, the presentations included:

- A paper co-authored by Dr. Alexander-Jackson and Dr. Virginia on "A Specific Type of Organism Cultivated from Malignancy: Bacteriology and Proposed Classification."

- A film by Dr. Alexander-Jackson and Dr. Virginia showing the *P. cryptocides* organisms living in blood samples of five terminal cancer patients.

- A paper by Dr. Irene Diller on "Experiments with Mammalian Tumor Isolates."

- A paper by Dr. Virginia's husband, Dr. A. M. Livingston, on "Toxic Fractions Obtained from Tumor Isolates and Related Clinical Implications."

- A paper by Florence Seibert, Ph.D., on "Morphological, Biological and Immunological Studies of Isolates from Tumors and Leukemic Bloods." (This was especially attention-getting, because Dr. Seibert, age seventy-four at the time of her participation in the section, had become famous by isolating purified protein derivative, thus making possible the isolation of the active substance of pure tuberculin. This work, done in the 1930s, is still the international standard for all the tuberculin made in the world. After retirement she volunteered for thirteen more years in programs examining the etiology of cancer.)

- A reading by Dr. Alexander-Jackson of her Rous paper, "Ultraviolet Spectrogramic Microscope Studies of Rous Sarcoma Virus Cultured in Cell-Free Medium."

Dr. Virginia's group was a huge success at the meeting, and their hypotheses about the microbial aspects of cancer were no longer ridiculed. Back at UCSD, they received more than 500 requests from all over the world for reprints of their papers and the articles published in the *Annals of the New York Academy of Sciences* (October 1970). Dr. Virginia at last felt satisfied that her lifetime of knowledge and experience was now on record in the leading science libraries of the world. This is why she just smiled when so many cancer physicians in later years kept asking her, "What scientific papers have you published?" In her feisty way, she usually replied that she had probably published more papers than all of them put together, if they would only take the trouble to look!

The Livingston Foundation Medical Center

Shortly after they returned home from New York, Dr. Virginia and her husband decided to open a clinic that would be available to cancer patients from all over the world. They hoped to treat the immune systems of such patients, bringing all the combined clinical and research experience of decades of work to bear on their disease. The case of her friend's husband, Dr. Ralph O., still hale and hearty years after he was declared terminal, encouraged their decision.

At the time of her death, the clinic was still open, providing immunotherapy to hundreds of new patients annually, and continuing a more than 90 percent rate of remissions in helping victims of cancer find the path to recovery and a normal, comfortable life span.

Afterward, the clinic, then called the Livingston Foundation Medical Center, changed somewhat and eventually closed in 1992. In 1977 Dr. Virginia had published *The Microbiology of Cancer: Compendium,* a collection of the above papers, independently published and copyrighted by the Livingston-Wheeler Medical Clinic. (Used copies are available online.)

However, also after her death, the treatment protocols for which she was roundly vilified began to develop further in research labs around the world until today not only are many of them accepted treatments, but some are actually preferred.

BCG? Now common in the treatment of bladder cancer and some other cancers.

Cruciferous veggies? There are immune-boosting broccoli sprouts actually available in your supermarket.

Autogenous vaccines? Many have been developed and several have already been FDA-approved.

Cancer caused by a bacterium? At least one has been identified as causing stomach cancer and others are being investigated.

It goes on and on. All of which validate my contention that Dr. Virginia Livingston-Wheeler was, indeed, "the woman who cured cancer."

A Final Note

This book could be 1,000 pages long and still be incomplete. That's how fast vaccine research is progressing in virtually every corner of the planet. Name a cancer—uterine, leukemia, melanoma, Hodgkin's, colon, glioma—and you'll find a hundred vaccine studies being conducted on potential new treatment protocols. There isn't time or space here to conduct an actual count, but there could very well be hundreds of Phase 3 (late-stage) trials, which compare new treatments with the best currently available treatment, going on at the Food and Drug Administration (FDA) as you read these words.

But I had to stop somewhere. The purpose of this book is not only to remind the public of Dr. Virginia's exalted position in the history of cancer research, but also to point out currently acceptable treatments that were once ridiculed when Dr. Virginia proposed them and to bring new hope and optimism to cancer victims everywhere—hope that Dr. Virginia tried in vain a generation ago to shout from the rooftops.

Even with all the new developments, it has been more than twenty years since we lost Dr. Virginia and her medical genius, but there are still researchers, doctors, and clinics around who provide and perform treatment protocols quite similar to hers. Some are called "alternative," but more often than not the protocols are a realistic combination of conventional therapies and so-called alternatives. Many are now called "integrative" treatments.

One such is the noted Issels Treatment Center in Santa Barbara, California, which also approximates the Livingston-Wheeler Clinic program. The late Josef M. Issels, M.D., was a leading pioneer of the conventional-plus-alternative approach to cancer, or what the treatment center calls "integrative immunotherapy." He founded a clinic in Germany in the early 1950s and apparently had such success in cancer remissions that all German insurance companies, including the equivalent of our Medicare, covered the treatment at Dr. Issels's hospital. In 1987, Dr. Issels retired from his activities in Germany and introduced the Issels Treatment, as it is called, to the United States. This integrative treatment uses all conventional protocols, as well as autogenous vaccines, diet, neutraceuticals (natural pharmaceuticals), monoclonal antibodies (gene-targeted therapy), and even the controversial laetrile.

Although Dr. Issels died in 1998, his wife, Ilse Marie Issels, and son, Christian N. Issels, N.D., continue to run the treatment center in Santa Barbara.

Cancer Support Services

There is an organization called CanHelp, founded by the aforementioned Patrick McGrady Jr., who was an old friend of mine. When Pat's father, Patrick Sr., a science writer/editor for the American Cancer Society (ACS) and the man who conceived and organized the ACS's Annual Science Writers Conference, contracted colon cancer and was unhappy with the treatment he received from the very organization he worked for, Pat immersed himself in cancer research in general and specific treatments in particular. In 1983 he founded CanHelp, an independent organization that refers cancer victims to the most efficacious alternative treatment protocols for their specific conditions. Pat died in 2003 of a blood clot following knee replacement surgery but the organization continues.

CanHelp investigates all so-called alternative treatments of cancer and visits practitioners and clinics around the country to evaluate their work; examine case history reports; and then recommends to clients which protocol is best suited to them.

The Livingston Foundation

A website has been created to give you the latest updates regarding the Livingston-Wheeler protocol and to preserve all of Dr. Virginia's writings, research, and discoveries. For further information on these and the availability of her vaccine, as well as the organizations cited above, see the following Resources section.

Resources

AUTOGENOUS VACCINE AND CIS-14 RETINOIC ACID

Bio Research Laboratories
John J. Majnarich, Ph.D.
2897 152nd Avenue NE
Redmond, WA 98052
Website: www.bioresearch.com
Email: info@bioresearch.com
Phone: (425) 869-4224 or (800) 886-3479

INTEGRATIVE IMMUNOTHERAPY CENTER

Issels Medical Center
1532 State Street
Santa Barbara, CA 93101
Phone: (805) 962-2126 or (888) 447-7357
Email: http://www.issels.com/questionnaire/
   questionnaire.aspx
Website: www.issels.com

RESOURCE ORGANIZATIONS

Can Help
P.O. Box 1678
Livingston, NJ 07039
Phone: 1-800-364-2341
Email: joan@canhelp.com
Website: www.canhelp.com

Livingston Foundation
Email: info@livingstonfoundation.com
Website: www.livingstinfoundation.com

Patient Advocates for Advanced Cancer Treatments (PAACT)
PO Box 141695
Grand Rapids, MI 49514
Phone: 616-453-1477
Email: paact@paactusa.org
Website: www.paactusa.org

FURTHER READING

Brennan, Richard. *Coronary? Cancer? God's Answer: Prevent It!* Irvine, CA: Harvest House Publishers, 1979.

Cantwell, Alan. *The Cancer Microbe: The Hidden Killer in Cancer, AIDS, and Other Immune Diseases.* Los Angeles: Aries Rising Press, 1990.

Glasser, Ronald. *The Body Is the Hero.* Glasgow, UK, William Collins Sons, 1976.

McGrady, Patrick. *The Savage Cell.* New York: Basic Books, 1964.

Siegel, Bernie. *Love, Medicine, and Miracles.* New York: William Morrow, 1986.

Index

About the Author

Edmond G. Addeo is a prolific author of non-fiction books on subjects ranging from sports to nutrition to social mores to teenage alcoholism. He has written three novels, has had two screenplays optioned, and has been a Los Angeles newspaperman and movie columnist, a science reporter and editor for McGraw-Hill World News and trade magazines, and an executive editor of a chain of community newspapers. As a freelancer, he has written articles on health subjects, travel and transportation, semiconductor technology, medical instrumentation, and celebrity profiles.

Addeo is a member of the Authors Guild. He lives with his wife in Mill Valley, California.